Nursing Delegation, Setting Priorities, and Making Patient Care Assignments

Second Edition

PATRICIA KELLY, RN, MSN
PROFESSOR EMERITUS
PURDUE UNIVERSITY CALUMET
HAMMOND, INDIANA
AND NCLEX-RN FACULTY
HOUSTON, TEXAS

MAUREEN T. MARTHALER, RN, MS
ASSOCIATE PROFESSOR OF NURSING
PURDUE UNIVERSITY CALUMET
HAMMOND, INDIANA

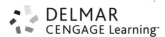
DELMAR
CENGAGE Learning™

Australia • Brazil • Japan • Korea • Mexico • Singapore • Spain • United Kingdom • United States

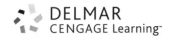
DELMAR
CENGAGE Learning™

Nursing Delegation, Setting Priorities, and Making Patient Care Assignments, Second Edition

Patricia Kelly, RN, MSN, and Maureen T. Marthaler, RN, MS

Vice president, Career and Professional Editorial: Dave Garza

Director of Learning Solutions: Matthew Kane

Executive Editor: Stephen Helba

Managing Editor: Marah Bellegarde

Editorial Assistant: Meghan Orvis

Vice President, Career and Professional Marketing: Jennifer McAvey

Marketing Director: Wendy Mapstone

Marketing Manager: Michelle McTighe

Marketing Coordinator: Scott Chrysler

Production Director: Carolyn Miller

Senior Art Director: Jack Pendleton

For product information and technology assistance, contact us at **Professional & Career Group Customer Support, 1-800-648-7450**

For Permission to use material from this text or product, submit all requests online at **cengage.com/permissions**. Further permissions questions can be e-mailed to **permissionrequest@cengage.com.**

Library of Congress Control Number: 2010922043

ISBN-13: 978-1-4354-8178-7

ISBN-10: 1-4354-8178-X

Delmar
5 Maxwell Drive
Clifton Park, NY 12065-2919
USA

Cengage Learning products are represented in Canada by Nelson Education, Ltd.

For your lifelong learning solutions, visit **delmar.cengage.com.**

Visit our corporate website at **cengage.com.**

Printed in the United States of America
1 2 3 4 5 6 14 13 12 11 10

CONTENTS

CONTRIBUTORS

Crisamar Javellana-Anunciado, MSN, APRN, BG
Inpatient Diabetes Nurse Practitioner
Sharp Chula Vista Medical Center
Chuta Vista, California

Sister Kathleen Cain, OSF, JD
Attorney
Franciscan Legal Services
Baton Rouge, Louisiana

Paul Heidenthal, MS
Consultant
Austin, Texas

Sharon Little-Stoetzel, RN, MS
Associate Professor of Nursing
Graceland University
Independence, Missouri

Patsy Maloney, RN, BC, EdD, MSN, MA, CNAA
Associate Professor/Director
Continuing Nursing Education
Pacific Lutheran University
Tacoma, Washington

Richard J. Maloney, BS, MA, MAHRM, EdD
Principal
Policy Governance Associates
Tacoma, Washington

Judith W. Martin, RN, JD
Attorney
Franciscan Legal Services
Baton Rouge, Louisiana

Terry W. Miller, PhD, RN
Dean and Professor
Pacific Lutheran University
School of Nursing
Tacoma, Washington

Robyn Pozza-Dollar, JD
Attorney
Cambridge, Massachusetts

Chad S. Priest, RN, BSN, JD
Attorney
Baker and Daniels, LLP
Adjunct Lecturer
Indiana University School of Nursing
Indianapolis, Indiana

Jacklyn Ludwig Ruthman, PhD, RN
Associate Professor
Bradley University
Peoria, Illinois

PREFACE

Nursing Delegation, Setting Priorities, and Making Patient Care Assignments, second edition, is designed to help nurses and nursing students develop the knowledge, skill, and competency to delegate nursing care quickly, efficiently, and safely, as well as to prepare for the National Council of State Boards of Nursing Licensure Examination for Registered Nurses (NCLEX-RN). The book is written primarily by two nursing authors with contributions from nurse faculty, nurse administrators, nurse managers, and nurse lawyers. These contributors hail from various areas of the United States, such as Illinois, Indiana, Massachusetts, Louisiana, Texas, Washington, California, and Missouri.

This reference will educate nursing students about the delegation process and supply the practicing nurse with practical information about delegation. In developing this book, we have integrated information from dozens of articles and books in nursing, health care, medicine, business, and the social sciences.

Safe delegation is critically important to nurses and patients. In the 1960s, nurse educators emphasized clinical skills and total patient care nursing, with the nurse managing the care of a few patients. Unfortunately, skill in delegation was not emphasized, and a generation of nurses was educated with very little knowledge about or practical experience with delegation. The recent nursing shortage has highlighted the need to change this. This book discusses the importance of nursing delegation as one of the skills a nurse needs to provide quality patient care. A List of Patient Descriptions appears before Chapter One; some of the patients are included in scenarios throughout the book to build knowledge and critical thinking skills. An assignment sheet is also included with the List of Patient Descriptions.

Each chapter discusses the latest information relevant to its specific topic. Chapters contain case studies, nursing or health care quotes, interviews, exercises, and evidence from the literature, all designed to enhance the reader's learning. Within each chapter, various points of view are presented through interviews with staff nurses, nursing administrators, physicians, and others. At the end of each chapter, there are web exercises, NCLEX-style review questions, skills activities, references, and suggested readings.

ORGANIZATION

Nursing Delegation, Setting Priorities, and Making Patient Care Assignments, second edition, consists of six chapters. These six chapters provide knowledge for beginning nurses to build skill and competency in delegating, setting priorities, and making patient care assignments in today's health care environment. This knowledge is also tested on the NCLEX-RN licensure examination. The chapters are arranged as follows:

Chapter One introduces the concept of delegation and applies it to nursing care of patients. Concepts of assignment, supervision, accountability, authority, responsibility, critical thinking, and decision making, as well as organizational responsibility for patient care, the chain of command, and Benner's Novice to Expert Model, are discussed.

Chapter Two covers the National Council of State Boards of Nursing Delegation Decision-Making Tree, the Five Rights of Delegation, principles of delegation, the role of State Boards of Nursing in delegation, sources of power, and delegation of responsibilities to health care team members. The National Council of State Boards of Nursing Tree highlights the elements of decision making that the nurse uses in delegating care. The Five Rights of Delegation emphasize elements the nurse uses to maintain safety for patients when delegating care. Power is explored as an important requirement for the nurse in developing delegation ability.

Chapter Three discusses effective communication. Nurses need effective communication skills to work with patients and health care team members of different cultures. The need for safe delegation emphasizes the importance of clear communication even more. This chapter also discusses the professional role of the nurse, potential barriers to communication, and the Myers-Briggs Personality Types. Workplace communication on a team involving crew resource management and SBARR is also discussed.

Chapter Four discusses time management, setting priorities, and making patient care assignments. Nurses use time management and priority-setting skills when delegating care. The nurse constantly assesses, evaluates, and re-assesses and re-evaluates patient care and safety when delegating care. The nurse identifies time wasters, learns to use time well, makes efficient patient handoff reports, and makes patient care assignments. Time management and priority setting assist with this process.

Chapter Five discusses legal aspects of patient care and delegation. The nurse considers legal aspects of delegating patient care and maintains patient safety with ethical behavior by avoiding common malpractice areas. This chapter discusses malpractice cases and identifies a nursing checklist to decrease the risk of liability.

Chapter Six discusses the NCLEX-RN examination. Samples of test questions, predictors of success, and elements of testing are included. A plan for your NCLEX-RN review, testing tips, and a brief medication review are also provided.

The book uses tables, figures, and photographs to engage learners and enhance their knowledge development. These features provide visual reinforcement of concepts such as delegation, communication, time management, setting priorities, the legal aspects of nursing, and preparation for NCLEX-RN.

CHAPTER FEATURES

The chapters include several features that provide the reader with a consistent format for learning and an assortment of resources for understanding and applying the information presented here.

These features include:

- A photo that begins each chapter and establishes the visual background for the reader's approach to the chapter.
- Quotes from a nursing or health care leader.

- **Real World Interview** boxes, which demonstrate various points of view on a given topic.
- **Keep Your Patients Safe** activities, which present a scenario and encourage the nurse to think critically to arrive at the best solution to maintain patient safety.
- **Review Questions,** written in NCLEX style, that test the reader's knowledge of important content.
- **Apply Your Skills** activities, which encourage the reader to build on the chapter content by applying the information to nursing activities.
- **Case Studies,** which encourage readers to think critically about how to apply chapter content to the workplace and other "real world" situations. Case Studies provide reinforcement of key delegation skills.
- **Exploring the Web** activities, which guide the reader by providing Internet addresses for the latest information related to the book's content.
- **Evidence from the Literature** applications, which link current literature to practice.
- References, which are the key to finding sources for the material presented in the book.
- Suggested Readings, which help the reader find additional information concerning the topics covered in the book.
- Glossary terms in **bold** type throughout each chapter. The glossary is designed to encourage understanding of new terms presented in the chapters; a complete Glossary appears at the end of the book.
- Tables and figures, which appear throughout the book and provide convenient information for the reader's reference.
- A list of patient descriptions before Chapter One, which is referenced in scenarios throughout the book to build critical-thinking and decision-making skills.

RESOURCES

A new **Online Companion** accompanies the second edition of this book and is available free of charge to users of the text. This valuable tool includes an **Answer Key** with suggested responses for the Opening Scenarios, Keep Your Patients Safe, Case Studies, Review Questions, and Apply Your Skills activities from the book. Also included for instructors are lecture slides created in **PowerPoint®**, and a **Computerized Test Bank**. Access the online companion at: http://www.delmarlearning.com/companions.

ACKNOWLEDGMENTS

Many people must work together to produce any book. A book such as this requires much effort and coordination of many people with various areas of expertise. I would like to thank all of the contributors for their time and effort in sharing their knowledge gained through years of experience in clinical, academic, and legal settings. I thank the reviewers for their time spent critically reviewing the manuscript and providing the valuable comments that have enhanced this book.

I would like to acknowledge and sincerely thank the team at Delmar Cengage Learning who have worked to make this book a reality. Elisabeth Williams is a great person who has worked tirelessly and brought knowledge, guidance, humor, and attention to keep me motivated and on track throughout the project.

Special thanks to my co-author, Maureen T. Marthaler, as we finish this second edition. Maureen is a pleasure to work with. Thanks also to Robyn Pozza-Dollar, who developed many of the legal tables in Chapter Five. Thanks also to Jo Reidy, Mercy Medical Center, Chicago, Illinois; Corinne Haviley, Northwestern Medical Center, Chicago, Illinois; and Dawn Moeller, Good Shepherd Medical Center, Barrington, Illinois, for their help in arranging some of the photographs for the book.

SPECIAL THANKS

A special thank you goes to my Aunt Pat Kelly, who encouraged me to start writing books. Special thanks also go to my parents, Ed and Jean Kelly; my sisters, Tessie Dybel and Kathy Milch; Aunt Verna and Uncle Archie Payne; Aunt Pat and Uncle Bill Kelly; my nieces, Natalie Bevil, Melissa Arredondo, and Stacey Milch; my nephew, John Milch; my grand nephew, Brock Bevil; my grand niece, Reese Bevil; nephews-in-law, Tracy Bevil and Peter Arredondo. Thanks also to my dear friends, Patricia Wojcik, Dolores Wynen, Florence Lebryk, and Lee McGuan, who have supported me through this book and most of my life. Special thanks to my wonderful nursing friends, Zenaida Corpuz, Dr. Mary Elaine Koren, Dr. Barbara Mudloff, Dr. Patricia Padjen, Jane McKeon, and especially to Gerri Kane, Janice Klepitch, Sylvia Komyatte, Julie Martini, Judy Rau, Anna Fizer, Trudy Keilman Walters, Judy Ilijanich, Ivy Schmude, Lillian Rau, Mary Kay Moredich, and others who have supported me throughout this book and during our 40 years together as nurses. Special thanks to my faculty mentors, Dr. Imogene King, Dr. Joyce Ellis, and Nancy Weber. Thanks also to Jane Woodruff for all of the computer support, and Eleanor DiAngelo and Joan Fox for their support during the review of this second edition.

ABOUT THE AUTHORS

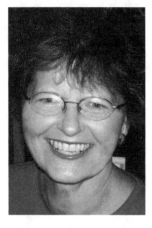

Patricia Kelly earned a Diploma in Nursing from St. Margaret Hospital School of Nursing in Hammond, Indiana; a baccalaureate in nursing from DePaul University in Chicago, Illinois; and a master's degree in nursing from Loyola University in Chicago, Illinois. She has worked as a staff nurse and as a school nurse. Pat has traveled extensively, teaching conferences for the Joint Commission. She was director of quality assurance for nursing at the University of Chicago Hospitals and Clinics in Chicago, Illinois.

Pat has taught at Wesley-Passavant School of Nursing, Chicago State University, and Purdue University Calumet in Hammond, Indiana. She is Professor Emeritus, Purdue University Calumet, Hammond, Indiana. Pat has taught fundamentals of nursing, adult nursing, nursing leadership and management, nursing issues, nursing trends, and legal aspects of nursing. She has taught nursing conferences on quality improvement in almost every state in the United States, as well as in Puerto Rico and Canada. Pat also teaches NCLEX-RN reviews nationally with Evolve NCLEX-RN Review and Testing, Houston, Texas, and is a member of Sigma Theta Tau and the American Nurses Association. She is listed in *Who's Who in American Nursing, 2000 Notable American Women*, and the *International Who's Who of Professional and Business Women*.

Pat has served on the Board of Directors of Tri City Mental Health Center, St. Anthony's Home, and Mosby's Quality Connection. She is the editor and author of *Nursing Leadership & Management*, Delmar Cengage Learning, 2003; *Essentials of Nursing Leadership & Management*, Delmar Cengage Learning, 2004; *Nursing Leadership & Management*, second edition, Delmar Cengage Learning, 2008; and *Essentials of Nursing Leadership & Management*, second edition, Delmar Cengage Learning, 2010. She also contributed a chapter entitled "Preparing the Undergraduate Student and Faculty to Use Quality Improvement in Practice" to *Improving Quality*, second edition, by Claire Gavin Meisenheimer, Aspen, 1997. She contributed a chapter entitled "Obstructive Lung Disease" to *Adult Health Nursing* by Rick Daniels, Delmar Cengage Learning, 2009. Pat has written several articles, including "Chest X-Ray Interpretation," and many articles on quality improvement. Pat is a disaster volunteer for the American Red Cross and has volunteered on health care trips to Nicaraugua, as well as at a free health clinic and at a church food pantry in Chicago, Illinois. Throughout much of her career, she has taught nursing at the university level and has continued to work part-time as a staff nurse in the Emergency Department. This has allowed her to wear several hats and see nursing from many points of view. Pat has been licensed and has worked in many states over her career, including Indiana, Illinois, Wisconsin, Oklahoma, New York, and Pennsylvania. Pat currently lives in Chicago, Illinois, and can be reached at patkelly777@aol.com.

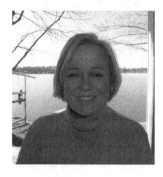

Maureen T. Marthaler earned a baccalaureate degree from Lewis University in Romeoville, Illinois, and a master's degree in nursing education from DePaul University in Chicago. She has taught at Prairie State College in Chicago Heights, Illinois. Currently, Maureen is an associate professor at Purdue University Calumet in Hammond, Indiana. Maureen has taught fundamentals of nursing, adult nursing, nursing leadership and management, freshman experience for nurses, pathophysiology, concepts or role development, RN refresher, and critical care nursing. She has taught at nursing conferences on various neurological conditions, such as neurological assessment, seizures, Guillain-Barre, Parkinson Disease, and blood gas interpretation. Maureen has also taught NCLEX reviews nationally. She is a member of Mu Omega Chapter of Sigma Theta Tau, National League for Nursing, and National Association of Clinical Specialists.

Maureen contributed a chapter on "Delegation of Patient Care" to the Patricia Kelly textbook, *Nursing Leadership & Management,* second edition, published by Delmar Cengage Learning in 2008. Her most recent publications include "Decompressive Hemicraniectomy with Duraplasty: A Treatment for Large-Volume Ischemic Stroke" in *The Journal of Neuroscience Nursing,* August 2005; and "End-of-Life Care: Practical Tips" in *Dimensions of Critical Care Nursing,* September/October 2005. She has traveled to Romania and assisted a nursing school there with curriculum development. Throughout her career, she has continued to practice part-time as a registered nurse in critical care at Metro South Hospital in Blue Island, Illinois.

Maureen has been licensed as an RN for more than 30 years. She is married to David, her wonderful husband and the father of their two sons, Luke, 21, and Jake, 19. They live in Crete, Illinois. Maureen can be reached via e-mail at Maureen@calumet.purdue.edu.

LIST OF PATIENT DESCRIPTIONS

The list below provides information about a group of patients. Some of the patients are referenced in scenarios throughout the book to help readers build critical-thinking and decision-making skills. Other patients are included for readers' use in making assignments; an assignment sheet is also included on page xiv.

Patient List		
Name	**Age**	**Patient Description**
Adult Patients		
Max Muench	27	Newly diagnosed with acquired immune deficiency syndrome (AIDS), has left lower lobe pneumonia
Michael Gray	61	Acute congestive heart failure (CHF), diabetic. Patient ran out of medications a week ago, diet and insulin instructions needed, cardiac rehabilitation, weigh daily
Susan Collier	92	New right hip fracture, in Bucks traction
Leona Glusak	89	Cerebrovascular accident (CVA) with right side paralysis this admission, transferred from ICU two days ago, vital signs, need to arrange home care
Nirmala Joseph	48	Acute cholelithiasis, confirmed by ultrasound
David Welch	41	Acute unstable angina, cardiac catheterization scheduled
Sylvia Thomas	60	Two days post intentional overdose (suicide attempt), sitter, cardiac monitor
Terry Summer	70	Hypertensive crisis, transferred from ICU yesterday (in ICU three days), BP now 180/102

Ramona Marriott	21	Acute asthma attack, wheezing, O2, Albuterol nebulizer, IV KVO
Jerry Williams	17	Sickle cell crisis, acute pain, IV, push fluids
Ed Moore	70	Acute ascites, history of alcohol abuse, IV
Pediatric Patients		
Irma Suria	6	Fever of unknown origin, temp 104
Malcolm Erickson	13	Acute congestive heart failure, three days post heart valve repair
Stewart Biggos	10	New onset diabetes mellitus, needs teaching
Reese Keating	3	MVA, new pneumothorax, chest tube, stable, parents at bedside
Brock Arredondo	8	Down Syndrome, bedfast, pneumonia, new trach, O2, IV, parents at bedside
Maria O'Connor	5	Wilm's Tumor, post-op one day, check voiding, IV
Maternal Child Patients		
Tess Dybel	22	One day post vaginal delivery, infant rooming in
Barbara Mudloff	23	Two days post C-section, ambulatory, infant rooming in
Lakeisha Soffey	17	One day postpartum, wants to give baby up for adoption
Jerry Dybel	Newborn	One day old
Jack Mudloff	Newborn	Two days old
Sara Soffey	Newborn	One day old, mother wants to give baby up for adoption
Mental Health Patients		
Ted Sorenson	19	Bipolar, very manic and pacing today
Jane Michaels	35	Schizophrenia, delusions
Joe Delray	27	Depression, attempted suicide/hanging, monitor closely

ASSIGNMENT SHEET

Unit _____

Date _____
Shift _____
Charge nurse _____
Breaks/Lunch _____
RNs _____
_____

LPN/LVNs _____
_____

NAP _____
_____

Notify RN immediately if:
T   <97 or >100
P   <60 or >110
R   <12 or >24
SBP <90 or >160
DBP <60 or >100
BS <70 or >200
Pulse oximetry <95%
Urine output < 30 cc/hour or
        240 cc/8hours

Notify RN one hour prior to
end of shift:
I&O
Patient goal achievement

Narcotic Count _____
Glucometer Calibration _____
Pass Water _____
Stock Linen _____
Code Cart _____
Medication refrigerator temperature check _____
Other _____

Room	Patient	Staff	A.M./P.M. Care	Weight I&O	IV	Activity	Glucometer	Tests	NPO	Comments

Room	Patient	Staff	A.M./P.M. Care	Weight I&O	IV	Activity	Glucometer	Tests	NPO	Comments

CHAPTER 1

Concept of Delegation

Maureen T. Marthaler, Sharon Little-Stoetzel,
Patricia Kelly

Both the
American
Nurses
Association and
state nursing
regulatory
bodies have
principles
specific to
delegation that
can assist the
chief nursing
officer in
fulfilling the
obligation of
accountability
for the provision
of safe nursing
care.
—Randall
   Hudspeth, 2007

OBJECTIVES

Upon completion of this chapter, the reader should be able to:

1. Discuss delegation.

2. Discuss overarching principles of delegation related to the organization and the nurse.

3. Define concepts of delegation, assignment, supervision, accountability, authority, and responsibility.

4. Review assignment sheets.

5. Compare direct and indirect delegation.

6. Review a health care organization's accountability for delegation.

7. Review the chain of command.

8. Identify elements of critical thinking and decision making.

9. Examine Benner's Model of Novice to Expert.

Sue Collier, a patient admitted with a right hip fracture and in Buck's traction, put the nurse call light on. The nurse answered the call light and placed the patient on the bed pan. The nurse told the nursing assistive personnel (NAP) that the patient was on the bed pan. Additionally, the nurse told the NAP that a urine sample was needed when the patient was taken off the bed pan. The NAP brought the urine sample to the nurse after taking the patient off the bed pan. Half an hour later, the nurse went into the patient's room and found the patient complaining of excruciating pain. The nurse checked the traction and found the weights on the floor. The NAP had removed the patient's weights before obtaining the urine sample and had failed to replace them.

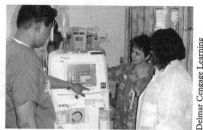

Who is responsible for the patient's traction weights being on the floor?

How could this situation have been prevented?

The nurse is responsible and accountable for individual nursing practice and determines the appropriate delegation of tasks consistent with the nurse's obligation to provide optimum patient care. The number one priority for nurses is to deliver safe patient care. To ensure that this responsibility is met, nurses are accountable under the scope and standards of nursing practice for patient care delivered by both themselves and other personnel under their supervision. These personnel may include other registered nurses (RNs), licensed practical/vocational nurses (LPN/LVNs), and nursing assistive personnel (NAP). "NAP" is an umbrella term applied to many categories of unlicensed assistive personnel, such as nurse aides, nurse technicians, patient care technicians, nurse support personnel, nurse extenders, personal care attendants, unit assistants, nursing assistants, and other non-licensed personnel. NAP are trained to function in an assistive role to the RN in providing patient care activities as delegated by the nurse. Note that in some states, health care assistive personnel are certified in some areas, as in the case of medication assistant-certified (MA-C) personnel.

This chapter will discuss the concepts of delegation, assignment, supervision, accountability, authority, and responsibility. It will also discuss Benner's Model of Novice to Expert, types of delegation, obstacles to delegation, organizational responsibility for delegation, the chain of command, and concepts of critical thinking and decision making.

PERSPECTIVES ON DELEGATION

Florence Nightingale is quoted as saying, "But then again to look to all these things yourself does not mean to do them yourself. . . . But can you not insure that it is done when not done by yourself?" (Nightingale, 1859). Nursing delegation was discussed by Nightingale in the 1800s and has continued to evolve since then. Delegation is needed because of the advent of cost containment, the shortage of nurses, increases in patient acuity levels, an elderly chronic population, and advances in health care technology.

Delegation is the transfer of responsibility for the performance of a task from one individual to another while retaining accountability for the outcome (American Nurses Association, 2005b) (www.safestaffing saveslives.org). In 2005, both the American Nurses Association (ANA) and the National Council of State Boards of Nursing (NCSBN) adopted papers on delegation and included them as attachments to a Joint Statement on Delegation, available at www.ncsbn.org. The Joint Statement's two attachments are the ANA Principles of Delegation and the NCSBN Decision Tree–Delegation to Nursing Assistive Personnel.

Note that state nurse practice acts define the legal parameters for nursing practice. Most states authorize RNs to delegate, and the nursing profession determines the scope of nursing practice (ANA and NCSBN, 2006). There is a need for competent, appropriately supervised NAP in the delivery of affordable, quality health care. The nursing profession defines and supervises the education, training, and utilization of all NAP involved in providing direct patient care.

PRINCIPLES

All decisions related to delegation are based on the fundamental principles of protection of the health, safety, and welfare of the public. There are overarching principles of delegation, nurse-related principles of delegation, and organization-related principles of delegation. Overarching principles of delegation include such elements as the idea that the nursing profession determines the scope of nursing practice. The nursing profession also takes responsibility and accountability for the provision of nursing practice (ANA, 2005b). Nursing-related principles include elements such as the idea that the RN may delegate elements of care but not the nursing process itself. RNs monitor organizational policies, procedures, and position descriptions to ensure there is no violation of the Nurse Practice Act, working with the state board of nursing, as necessary. Chief nursing officers (CNOs) are responsible for establishing systems to assess, monitor, verify, and communicate ongoing competence requirements in areas related to delegation, both for RNs and delegates (ANA, 2005b).

Organization-related principles guiding nursing delegation include such elements as the organization is accountable for documenting staff competence, developing organizational policies on delegation, and allocating resources to ensure safe staffing (ANA, 2005b). See Figure 1-1.

REAL WORLD INTERVIEW

As a pediatric nurse, I delegate several tasks to NAP including: stocking supplies, giving baths, changing linen, feeding patients, taking vital signs, orienting parents to the unit's layout (refrigerator, phone, sleep area, shower room, etc.), and picking up medications from the pharmacy. When I delegate to NAP, I always double-check that the job was done correctly and make sure it was done in a timely manner and to the patient's liking.

Beth Michalesko, RN
St. John, Indiana

As health care changes and RN shortages demand adaptations in the manner that care is provided, RNs become responsible for the delegation of support services and care tasks through the supervision of increased numbers and types of NAP (Center for American Nurses, 2008). Delegating to personnel with different educational levels from a variety of educational programs requires nurses to be vigilant and ensure that safety is maintained for the patient. When delegating to all levels of nursing staff, RNs are accountable for the outcome of patient care. For example, when an RN delegates the process of ambulating a patient to NAP, the RN remains accountable for assessing the patient's ability to ambulate, assuring that the patient is ambulated according to standards, and helping the patient achieve a safe outcome, that is, preventing a fall. The RN must monitor the competency, education, and skill of NAP and the stability of the patient needing a delegated task. This monitoring is done initially and continues throughout the task. Thus, efficient delegation protects the patient.

ASSIGNMENT

Assignment is defined by both ANA and NCSBN (2006) as the distribution of work that each staff member is responsible for during a given shift or work period. The NCSBN uses the verb "assign" to describe those situations when a nurse directs an individual to do something the individual is already authorized to do (ANA and NCSBN, 2006).

Elements to Consider

- Federal, state, and local regulations and guidelines for practice, including the state nurse practice act
- Nursing professional standards
- Health care agency policy, procedure, and standards

- Job description of Registered Nurse, Licensed Practical Nurse/Licensed Vocational Nurse, Nursing Assistive Personnel
- Five Rights of Delegation
- Knowledge and skill of personnel

- Documented personnel competency, strengths, and weaknesses (select the right person for the right job)
- ANA principles for delegation, i.e., overarching principles, nurse-related principles, and organization-related principles*

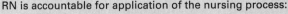

RN is accountable for application of the nursing process:
- Assessment and nursing judgment**
- Nursing diagnosis
- Planning care
- Implementation and teaching
RN delegates as appropriate.
RN retains accountability.
Note that LPN/LVNs and NAP are also responsible for their actions.***

RNs	LPN/LVNs	NAP
RNs assess, plan care, monitor, and evaluate all patients, especially complex, unstable patients with unpredictable outcomes.	LPN/LVNs care for stable patients with predictable outcomes. They work under the direction of the RN and are responsible for their actions within their scope of practice.	NAP assist the RNs and the LPN/LVNs and give technical care to stable patients with predictable outcomes and minimal potential for risk. They work under the direction of an RN and are responsible for their actions.
Administer medications, including IV push and IVPBs.	Gather patient data.	
Start and maintain IVs and blood transfusions.	Implement patient care.	Assist with activities of daily living.
	Maintain infection control.	
Perform sterile or specialized procedures, i.e., Foley catheter and nasogastric tube insertion,	Provide teaching from standard teaching plan.	Assist with bathing, grooming, and dressing.
	Depending on the state and with documented	Assist with toileting and bed making.

(continues)

Figure 1-1 Considerations in delegation. (Delmar Cengage Learning.)

RNs	LPN/LVNs	NAP
tracheostomy care, suture removal, and so on.	competency, may do the following:***	Ambulate, position, and transport.
Educate patient and family.	• Administer medications.	Feed and socialize with patient.
Maintain infection control.	• Perform sterile or specialized procedures, for example, Foley catheter and nasogastric tube insertion, tracheostomy care, suture removal, and so on.	Measure intake & output (I&O).
Administer cardiopulmonary resuscitation.		Document care.
Interpret and report laboratory findings.		Weigh patient.
Triage patients.	• Perform blood glucose monitoring.	Maintain infection control.
Prevent nurse-sensitive patient outcomes, for example, cardiac arrest, pneumonia, and so on.	• Administer CPR.	Depending on the state and with documented competency, may do the following:***
Monitor patient outcomes.	• Perform venipuncture and insert peripheral IVs, change IV bags for patients receiving IV therapy, and so on.	• Perform blood glucose monitoring.
		• Collect specimens.
		• Administer CPR.
		• Take vital signs.
		• Perform 12-lead EKGs.
		• Perform venipuncture for blood tests.

Evaluation
RN uses judgment and is responsible for evaluation of all patient care.

*www.nursingworld.org. search for ANA principles for delegation, 2005.
****Nursing judgment** is the process by which nurses come to understand the problems, issues, and concerns of patients, to attend to salient information, and respond to patient problems in concerned and involved ways. Judgment includes both conscious decision making and intuitive response (Benner, Tanner, & Chesla, 1996).
***Some variation from state to state and health care agency.

Figure 1-1 *(continued)*

For example, when an RN directs another RN to assess a patient, the second RN is already authorized to assess patients in the RN scope of practice. A 2003 survey of hospitals and individuals working in hospitals states, "Assignments and delegation of activities of care are based on the nurse's assessment of patient needs and are congruent with the caregiver's knowledge and skill" (American Organization of Nurse Executives, 2003). During a typical shift, patients range from those needing only occasional care to those requiring frequent care. The charge nurse makes out the assignment sheet taking into consideration the skill, knowledge, and judgment of the RNs, LPN/LVNs, and NAP. Assignments are given to staff who have the appropriate knowledge and skill to complete them. Assignments must always be within the legal scope of practice. Assignment sheets are used to identify patient care duties for RNs, LPN/LVNs, and NAP (Figure 1-2).

Decisions to delegate nursing tasks, functions, and activities are based on the needs of clients, the stability of client conditions, the complexity of the task, the predictability of the outcome, the available resources to meet those needs, and the judgment of the nurse (NCSBN, 1995). The RN uses critical thinking and is accountable for the appropriateness of delegated nursing tasks. Inappropriate delegation by the nurse and/or unauthorized performance of nursing tasks by NAP may lead to legal action against the nurse and/or NAP. A task delegated to NAP cannot be redelegated by NAP. When a nursing task is delegated, the task must be performed in accord with established standards of practice, policies, and procedures. The nurse who delegates retains accountability for the task delegated (NCSBN, 1995).

STANDARDS

Standards of practice, policies, and procedures are established by the nursing profession, the state nurse practice act, and the health care organization. Standards are written and used to guide both the provision and evaluation of patient care by RNs and NAP. When the RN delegates care to other members of the health care team, the RN must share the standards of practice, policies, and procedures with the other team members. These standards serve as guidelines and are the basis for evaluation of patient care given by the RN and all members of the health care team.

Note that there is a significant difference between delegating patient care to another RN and delegating patient care to an LPN/LVN or NAP. The work given to the RN, LPN/LVN, or NAP must fall within the individual's legal scope of practice. Experienced RNs are expected to work with minimal supervision of their nursing practice. The RN who gives patient care to another competent RN, who then assumes responsibility and accountability for that patient's care, does not have the same obligation to closely supervise that person's work as when the care is given to an LPN/LVN or NAP. The RN can give responsibility to the LPN/LVN or NAP, but the RN retains accountability for the patient's care. LPN/LVNs and NAP work under the direction of the RN.

Date _____

Unit _____

Shift _____

Charge nurse _____

RNs _____

Lunch/Breaks _____

LPN/LVNs _____

NAP _____

Lunch/Breaks _____

Notify RN immediately if:

*T   <97 or >100

*P   <60 or >110

*R   <12 or >24

*SBP <90 or >160

*DBP <60 or >100

*BS   <70 or >150

Pulse oximetry <95%

Room	Staff	IV, Tube Feeding	Foley, I&O, Drains, Weight	NPO	Activity	Glucometer Monitor	Lab and X-ray	Comments

Check Crash Cart _____ Pass Water _____

Glucometer Check _____ Stock Linen _____

Other _____

*T = Temperature   *R = Respirations   *DBP = Diastolic Blood Pressure

*P = Pulse   *SBP = Systolic Blood Pressure   *BS = Blood Sugar

Figure 1-2 Assignment sheet. (Delmar Cengage Learning.)

Patient care can properly be completed by an individual (such as another RN) who understands the assignment; has the necessary skill, knowledge, and judgment; and acts within the legal authority of the regulatory scope of practice. An example is a charge nurse assigning the care of four patients to a staff RN. The nurse making the assignment is accountable for his or her decision in making the assignment. It is inappropriate for the charge nurse to assign the total care of a complex patient to a new graduate nurse until the new graduate is completely oriented and prepared for the care of that patient. However, once the new staff nurse accepts the assignment, he or she will assume responsibility and accountability for the care of that patient. That individual is now practicing on the basis of his or her own credentials.

Certain actions may be given to an LPN/LVN in keeping with the scope of practice as designated by state regulation. If the LPN/LVN is certified in intravenous (IV) therapy, and the policy of the state and the employing institution permits LPN/LVNs to provide IV treatment, the RN should not have an inordinate duty to supervise the work once the LPN/LVN's skills in this area are demonstrated. Note that prior competency certification of the LPN/LVN may have been done through a skills day or through a competency validation. This competency validation may ensure that the LPN/LVN has been observed inserting an IV successfully three times under direct supervision of an RN in states where this practice by an LPN/LVN is allowed. The RN cannot give responsibility and accountability for total nursing care to NAP or LPN/LVNs, but the RN can delegate certain tasks to them in keeping with the state law, job description, knowledge base, and demonstrated competency of these individuals.

COMPETENCE

Competence is the ongoing ability of a nurse to integrate and apply the knowledge, skills, judgment, and personal attitudes required to practice safely and ethically in a designated role and setting (Canadian Nurses Association, 2004). Licensed nurse competence is built upon the knowledge gained in a nursing education program and during the experiences of practicing nursing. The nurse must know himself or herself first, including individual strengths and challenges; assess the match of his or her knowledge and experience with the requirements and context of a specific role and setting; gain additional knowledge as needed; and maintain all skills and abilities needed to provide safe nursing care. Competence requires the application of knowledge and the interpersonal, decision-making, and psychomotor skills expected for the practice role (NCSBN, 1995).

NAP competence is built upon formal training and assessment, orientation to specific settings and groups of patients, interpersonal and communication skills, and the experience of the NAP in assisting the nurse to provide safe nursing care.

Health care organizations require employees to demonstrate that they are competent to perform certain technical procedures and apply specific knowledge to safely care for patients. Written documentation of these competencies is maintained in the employee's personnel file. Most health care organizations require employees to undergo annual competency training for elements of care unique to their practice setting. Annual competency testing for RN, LPN/LVN, and NAP may include: patient safety, infection control, code blue, medication safety, IV skills, glucose testing, chain of command, HIPAA (Health Insurance Portability and Accountability Act) policies, and restraints.

KEEP YOUR PATIENTS SAFE 1-1

Complete the assignment sheet in Figure 1-2 using five adult hospitalized patients from the patient list in the front of this book. Choose assignments for the RN, LPN/LVN, and NAP and decide how you will delegate and assign the work.

SUPERVISION

NCSBN defines **supervision** as the provision of guidance or direction, oversight, evaluation, and follow-up by the licensed nurse for the accomplishment of a delegated nursing task by assistive personnel. ANA defines supervision as the active process of directing, guiding, and influencing the outcome of an individual's performance of a task. Both the NCSBN and ANA define supervision as the provision of guidance and oversight of a delegated nursing task (ANA and NCSBN, 2006). Supervision means personally observing a function or activity, providing leadership in the process of nursing care, delegating functions or activities while retaining accountability, and evaluating or determining that nursing care being provided is adequate and delivered appropriately (Marthaler, 2009). Supervision is generally categorized as direct (the nurse being physically present or immediately available while the activity is being performed) or indirect (the nurse has the ability to provide direction through various means of written and verbal communication).

A nurse who is supervising care should provide clear directions to his or her staff about what assignments are to be performed for a specific group of patients. The supervising nurse must identify when and how assignments are to be done and what information must be collected, as well as any patient-specific information. The nurse must identify what outcomes are expected and the time frame for reporting results. The nurse will monitor staff performance to ensure compliance with established standards of practice, policy, and procedure. The supervising nurse will obtain feedback from staff and patients and intervene, as necessary, to ensure quality nursing care and appropriate documentation.

Hansten and Jackson (2009) identify varying levels of supervision, which will be used as a base in regards to the frequency of periodic follow-up.

- Never-delegated tasks are parts of the nursing practice act that the nurse never delegates. Assessment, nursing diagnosis, planning, evaluation, and certain parts of the intervention are included in the never-delegate category.
- Unsupervised tasks occur when two RNs are working together. Neither needs follow-up unless the charge nurse sees the need to do so.
- Initial direction/periodic inspection is directly related to when the RN delegates a task, knowing staff capabilities in terms of competency to an unlicensed, newly licensed, or temporary RN.
- Continuous supervision is when the RN is not familiar with the individual's competency nor has a professional relationship with that individual.

ACCOUNTABILITY

Accountability is being responsible and answerable for actions or inactions of self or others in the context of delegation (NCSBN, 1995). The RN is accountable for the performance of tasks delegated to others, for tasks the nurse personally performs, and for the act of delegating activities to others. Licensed nurse accountability involves compliance with legal requirements as set forth in the jurisdiction's laws and rules governing nursing. The licensed nurse is also accountable for the quality of the nursing care provided; for recognizing limits, knowledge, and experience; and for planning for situations beyond the nurse's expertise (NCSBN, 1995). Licensed nurse accountability includes the preparedness and obligation to explain or justify to relevant others (including the regulatory authority) the related initial and ongoing judgments, intentions, decisions, actions, and omissions . . . and the consequences of those decisions, actions, and behaviors. Nurses are accountable for following their state nurse practice act, standards of professional practice, policies of their health care organization, and ethical-legal models of behavior. RNs are accountable for monitoring changes in a patient's status, noting and implementing treatment for human responses to illness, and assisting in the prevention of complications.

The RN assesses the patient; makes a nursing diagnosis; and develops, implements, and evaluates the patient's plan of care. The RN uses nursing judgment and monitors unstable patients with unpredictable outcomes. The monitoring of other, more stable patients cared for by the LPN/LVN and NAP may involve the RN's direct continuing presence, or the monitoring may be more intermittent. As stated by the AACN (2004), the delegation of direct and indirect patient care to other caregivers is reasonable, relevant, and practical. Nursing tasks that do not involve direct patient care can be reassigned more freely and carry fewer legal implications for RNs than delegation of direct nursing practice activities. The assessment, analysis, diagnosis, planning, teaching, and evaluation stages of the nursing process may not be delegated to NAP. Delegated activities usually fall within the implementation phase of the nursing process. When authority has been delegated and responsibility assumed, the delegate is then accountable for the delegated task. The accountability for the performance of the task becomes shared, because the delegator also remains accountable for the completion of the delegated task. Accountability for delegation also rests with the organization through allocating resources to ensure staffing, documenting competencies for all staff providing direct patient care, and ensuring access to information for those delegating patient care.

NAP and LPN/LVNs are also accountable to the RN. Accountability for the act of delegating involves the appropriate choice of person and activity. For example, an RN might delegate to NAP the authority to perform a certain task. If the RN has not determined in advance that the person understands the assignment and has the skills, knowledge, and judgment to fulfill the task, or the RN does not supervise the task completion and the NAP does not perform the task adequately, the RN would be accountable for this act of improper delegation.

AUTHORITY

Authority is the right to act or to command the action of others. Authority comes with the job and is required for a nurse to take action. The person to whom a task and authority have been delegated must be free to make decisions regarding the activities involved in performing that task. Without authority, the nurse cannot function to meet the needs of patients. Authority is commonly delegated to the nurse in the nurse's job description. See Figure 1-3.

Authority is based on each individual state's nurse practice act. If a nurse is in charge of a group of patients, the nurse must have the authority or the right to act or command the action of others. Note that there are

ALBANY MEDICAL CENTER
HOSPITAL PATIENT CARE SERVICES
Job Description

JOB TITLE: REGISTERED PROFESSIONAL NURSE

Exempt (Y/N): No	JOB CODE:
SALARY LEVEL: N25.1-4	DOT CODE:
SHIFT:	DIVISION: PATIENT CARE SVC
LOCATION: NURSING UNITS	DEPARTMENT:
EMPLOYEE NAME:	SUPERVISOR: NURSE MANAGER
PREPARED BY: AMY BALUCH	DATE: 03/22/XX
APPROVED BY:	DATE:

SUMMARY: The Registered Professional Nurse utilizes the nursing process to diagnose and treat human responses to actual or potential health problems. The New York State Nurse Practice Act and A.N.A. Code for Nurses with Interpretive Statements guide the practice of the Registered Professional Nurse. The primary responsibility of the Registered Professional Nurse as leader of the Patient Care Team is coordination of patient care through the continuum, education, and advocacy.

ESSENTIAL DUTIES AND RESPONSIBILITIES include the following. Other duties may be assigned.

—Performs an ongoing and systematic assessment, focusing on physiologic, psychologic, and cognitive status.

—Develops a goal-directed plan of care that is standards-based. Involves patient and/or significant other (S.O.) and health care team members in patient-care planning.

—Implements care through utilization and adherence to established standards that define the structure, process, and desired patient outcomes of nursing process.

—Evaluates effectiveness of care in progressing patients toward desired outcomes. Revises plan of care based on evaluation of outcomes.

—Demonstrates competency in knowledge base, skill level, and psychomotor skills.

—Demonstrates applied knowledge base in areas of structure standards, standards of care, protocols, and patient care resources/references. Practices in compliance with state and federal regulations.

(continues)

Figure 1-3 Job description. (Courtesy Albany Medical Center, Hospital Patient Care Services, job description for registered professional nurses, Albany, NY.)

—Demonstrates knowledge of Patient Bill of Rights by incorporating it into their practice.

—Demonstrates ability to identify, plan, implement and evaluate patient/S.O. education needs.

—Participates in development and attainment of unit and service patient care goals.

—Organizes and coordinates delivery of patient care in an efficient and cost effective manner.

—Documents the nursing process in a timely, accurate and complete manner, following established guidelines.

—Utilizes standards in applying the nursing process for the delivery of patient care.

—Participates in unit and service quality management activities.

—Demonstrates self-directed learning and participation in continuing education to meet own professional development.

—Participates in team development activities for unit and service.

—Demonstrates responsibility and accountability for professional standards and for own professional practice.

—Supports research and its implications for practice.

—Adheres to unit and human resource policies.

—Establishes and maintains direct, honest, and open professional relationships with all health care team members, patients, and significant others.

—Seeks guidance and direction for successful performance of self and team to meet patient care outcomes.

—Incorporates into practice an awareness of legal and risk management issues and their implications.

QUALIFICATION REQUIREMENTS: To perform this job successfully, an individual must be able to perform each essential duty satisfactorily. The requirements listed below are representative of the knowledge, skill, and/or ability required. Reasonable accommodations may be made to enable individuals with disabilities to perform the essential functions.

(continues)

Figure 1-3 *(continued)*

EDUCATION and/or EXPERIENCE: Graduate of an approved program in professional nursing. Must hold current New York State registration or possess a limited permit to practice in the State of New York.

LANGUAGE SKILLS: Ability to read and interpret documents such as safety rules and procedure manuals. Ability to document patient care on established forms. Ability to speak effectively to patients, family members, and other employees of organization.

MATHEMATICAL SKILLS: Ability to add, subtract, multiply, and divide in all units of measure, using whole numbers, common fractions, and decimals. Ability to compute rate, ratio, and percent.

REASONING ABILITY: Ability to identify problems, collect data, establish facts, and draw valid conclusions.

PHYSICAL DEMANDS: The physical demands described here are representative of those that must be met by an employee to successfully perform the essential functions of this job. Reasonable accommodations may be made to enable individuals with disabilities to perform the essential functions.

While performing the duties of this job, the employee is regularly required to stand; walk; use hands to probe, handle, or feel objects, tools, or controls; reach with hands and arms; and speak or hear. The employee is occasionally required to sit or stoop, kneel, or crouch.

The employee must regularly lift and/or move up to 100 pounds and frequently lift and/or move more than 100 pounds. Specific vision abilities required by this job include close vision, distance vision, peripheral vision, depth perception, and the ability to adjust focus.

WORK ENVIRONMENT: The work environment characteristics described here are representative of those an employee encounters while performing the essential functions of this job. Reasonable accommodations may be made to enable individuals with disabilities to perform the essential functions.

While performing the duties of this job, the employee is regularly exposed to bloodborne pathogens.

The noise level in the work environment is usually moderate.

rev. 9/95
rev. 6/96

Figure 1-3 *(continued)*

TABLE 1-1 *LEVELS OF AUTHORITY*	
Level	**Authority**
One	Delegate to collect data to simply find out the facts or assess the situation and report back.
Two	Delegate to collect data and report back to the RN.
Three	Delegate to assess the situation, make a recommendation, report back, and then implement the final RN recommendation.
Four	Delegate to carry out the task as the RN believes is appropriate.

Adapted from Motivation and Morale: Coin of the Realm, by S. H. Cox, 1997. Symposium conducted at Nursing Management Congress, Washington, DC.

four possible levels of authority to be used by the RN when delegating a task to another nurse (Cox, 1997). See Table 1-1.

An understanding of the level of authority at the time the task is delegated and the level of authority that is identified by the state nurse practice act and the health care agency's job description prevents each party from making inaccurate assumptions about authority for delegated assignments.

RESPONSIBILITY

Responsibility is the obligation involved when one accepts an assignment. The delegation process is not complete until the person who receives the assignment accepts it. Without this acceptance of obligation or responsibility, authority cannot be delegated. Further, if a person does not have the knowledge, skill, experience, or willingness needed to complete an assignment, it is inappropriate to accept responsibility for that assignment.

Once a person accepts responsibility, this responsibility is retained. For example, after the NAP's duty is performed, the NAP is responsible to report feedback to the nurse about the performance and outcome of the duty within a specified time frame. It is the NAP's responsibility to give a feedback report, and it is the RN's responsibility to follow up with ongoing supervision and evaluation of the NAP activities. The nurse transfers authority for the completion of a delegated task, but retains responsibility and accountability for monitoring the delegated task's outcome.

KEEP YOUR PATIENTS SAFE 1-2

The charge nurse assigned a nurse who recently passed the NCLEX to change the intravenous (IV) sites on two patients. Three days ago, the two nurses started new IV sites together. This was the first time the new nurse had started IV sites. Gathering the equipment needed for the assigned patient care, the new nurse walks down the hallway, thrilled to have been given this opportunity.

Does the charge nurse have the authority to allow the new nurse to start IVs? What is the rationale for your answer?

DELEGATED ACTIVITIES

The decision whether or not to delegate uses the RN's judgment concerning the condition of the patient; the competence, knowledge, and skill of the nursing team members; and the degree of supervision that will be required of the RN if a task is delegated. The RN delegates only those tasks for which he or she believes a NAP has the knowledge and skill to perform, taking into consideration training, culture, experience, and the health care organization's policies and procedures. The RN individualizes communication regarding the delegation to NAP and patient situation. The communication should be clear, concise, correct, and complete (Hansten and Jackson, 2009). The RN verifies comprehension with the NAP and assures that the NAP accepts the delegation. The NAP is then also answerable for his or her actions and behavior and the responsibility that accompanies them (NCSBN, 2005). Communication between the RN and NAP must be a two-way process. NAP should have the opportunity to ask questions and seek clarification of delegated tasks.

The RN assures that all communication is culturally appropriate and that the person receiving it is treated respectfully. Note that there is both individual accountability and organizational accountability for delegation. It is inappropriate for employers or others to require nurses to delegate when, in the nurse's professional judgment, delegation is unsafe and not in the patient's best interest. In those instances, the nurse should act as the patient's advocate and take appropriate action to ensure provision of safe nursing care. If the nurse determines that delegation may not appropriately take place, but nevertheless delegates as directed, the nurse may be disciplined by the Board of Nursing (NCSBN, 1995). There are two types of patient care activities that may be delegated: direct and indirect.

DIRECT PATIENT CARE

Direct patient care activities include activities that assist the patient with feeding, drinking, ambulating, grooming, toileting, dressing, and socializing. A direct patient care activity may also involve reporting and documenting care related to the activity. This data is reported to the RN, who uses the information to make a clinical judgment about patient care. Activities delegated to NAP do not include health counseling or teaching or activities that require independent, specialized nursing knowledge, skill, or judgment.

INDIRECT PATIENT CARE

Indirect patient care activities are often necessary to support patients and their environment, and only incidentally involve direct patient contact. These activities are often designated "unit routines" and assist in providing a clean, efficient, and safe patient care milieu. These activities do not require the special training or skills that direct patient care activities require of NAP. Housekeeping, clerical work, stocking supplies, and other tasks similar to these are examples of indirect patient care.

UNDERDELEGATION

Individuals in a new nursing role often underdelegate. Believing that older, more experienced staff may resent having someone new delegate to them, new nurses may simply avoid delegation. The new nurse may seek approval from other staff members by demonstrating capability to complete all assigned duties without assistance, or without delegating.

New nurses can become frustrated and overwhelmed if they fail to delegate properly. They may also fail to delegate certain tasks to the appropriate person. Perfectionism and refusal to allow mistakes can overwhelm a new nurse. More experienced staff members can help new nurses by intervening early and assisting in the delegation process, by clarifying roles and responsibilities, and by expressing willingness to work with the new RN.

OVERDELEGATION

Overdelegation of duties can place the patient at risk. The reasons for overdelegation are numerous. Personnel may feel uncomfortable performing duties that are unfamiliar to them, and they may depend too much on others. They may be unorganized or inclined to either avoid responsibility or immerse themselves in paperwork. Overdelegation leads to delegating

TABLE 1-2
OBSTACLES TO DELEGATION

- Fear of being disliked
- Inability to give up control of the situation
- Inability to determine what to delegate and to whom
- Past experience with delegation that did not turn out well
- Lack of confidence to move beyond being a novice nurse
- Tendency to isolate oneself and choosing to complete all tasks alone
- Lack of confidence in delegating to staff that were previously one's peers
- Inability to prioritize using Maslow's Hierarchy of Needs and the Nursing Process
- Thinking of oneself as the only one who can complete a task the way it is supposed to be done
- Inability to develop working relationships with other team members
- Lack of knowledge of the capabilities of staff, including their competency, skill, experience, level of education, job description, and so on
- Fear of being viewed as being unable to care for patients independently
- Fear of staff refusing to carry out delegated tasks
- Lack of administrative support
- Poor communication skills

duties to personnel who are not educated for the tasks, such as LPN/LVNs and NAP. Delegating duties that are inappropriate for personnel to perform because they have been inadequately educated is dangerous and against state nurse practice acts. Overdelegating duties can overwork some personnel and underwork others, creating obstacles to delegation. See Table 1-2.

ORGANIZATIONAL ACCOUNTABILITY FOR DELEGATION

Organizational accountability for delegation includes providing sufficient resources, including sufficient staffing with an appropriate staff mix; documenting competencies for all staff providing direct patient care; ensuring that the RN has access to competency information for the staff to whom the RN is delegating care; providing opportunities for continuing staff development; creating an environment conducive to teamwork, collaboration, and patient-centered care; and developing organizational policies on delegation with the active participation of all nurses. These policies on delegation must acknowledge that delegation is a professional nursing right and responsibility. Note that CNOs are accountable for establishing systems to assess, monitor, verify, and communicate ongoing competency requirements in areas related to delegation, both for RNs and for delegates (ANA and NCSBN, 2006). The organization is accountable for delegation through the allocation of resources to ensure sufficient staffing so that the RN can delegate appropriately. The organization must also ensure that the education needs of nurses are met through the implementation of a system that allows for nurse input. Organizations fulfill their responsibility to staff and patients by developing these elements and defining a clear chain of command. See Table 1-3.

TABLE 1-3

ORGANIZATIONAL ELEMENTS NEEDED FOR EFFICIENT DELEGATION

- Follow professional standards for education, licensure, and competency in all hiring decisions, orientation, and ongoing continuing education programs.
- Maintain adequate staffing.
- Have clear job descriptions and ongoing licensing and credentialing policies for RNs, MDs, LPN/LVNs, NAP, and other health care staff. The organization must ensure that all staff members are safe, competent practitioners before assigning them to patient care. Orient staff to their duties, chain of command, and the job descriptions of RN, LPN/LVN, and NAP.
- Facilitate clinical and educational specialty certification and credentialing of all health care practitioners and staff.
- Provide standards for ongoing supervision and periodic licensure/competency verification and evaluation of all staff.
- Provide access to professional health care standards, policies, procedures, library, Internet, and medication information with unit availability and efficient library and Internet access.
- Facilitate regular evidence-based reviews of critical standards, policies, and procedures.
- Have clear policies and procedures for delegation and chain of command reporting lines for all staff from RN to charge nurse to nurse manager to nurse executive and, as appropriate, to risk management, the hospital ethics committee, the hospital administrator, nursing and medical practitioners, the chief of the medical staff, the board of directors, the State Licensing Board for Nursing and Medicine, and the Joint Commission.
- Provide administrative support for supervisors and staff who delegate, assign, monitor, and evaluate patient care.
- Clarify health care provider accountability. For example, if a medical or nursing practitioner or physician assistant delegates a nursing task to

(continues)

Table 1-3 *(continued)*

NAP, the health care provider is responsible for monitoring that care delivery. This must be spelled out in hospital policy. If the RN notes that NAP is doing something incorrectly, the RN has a duty to intervene and to notify the ordering health care provider of the incident.

- Consider need to develop a shared governance model of nursing practice to encourage active participation by all nurses in decision-making and delegation standards.
- The RN always has an independent responsibility to protect patient safety. Blindly relying on another nursing or health care provider is not permissible for the RN.
- Provide education and standards for regular RN evaluation of NAP and LPN/LVN, and reinforce the need for NAP and LPN/LVN accountability to the RN. RNs must delegate and supervise. They cannot abdicate this professional responsibility.
- Develop a physical, mental, and verbal "No Abuse" policy to be followed by all professional and nonprofessional health care staff. Follow up on any problems.
- Consider applying for magnet status for your facility. This status is awarded by the American Nurses Credentialing Center to health care agencies that have worked to improve nursing care, including the empowering of nursing decision making and delegation in clinical practice (www.nursingworld.org).
- Monitor patient outcomes, including nurse-sensitive outcomes, staffing ratios, and other quality indicators. Develop ongoing clinical quality improvement practices. Benchmark with national groups.
- Maintain ongoing monitoring of incident reports, sentinel events, and other elements of risk management and performance improvement of the process and outcome of patient care.
- Develop systematic, error-proof systems for medication administration that ensure the six "rights" of medication administration, that is, the right patient, right medication, right dose, right time, right route, and right documentation. Develop safe computerized order-entry systems.
- Provide documentation of routine maintenance for all patient care equipment.
- Attain the JC Patient Safety Goals (www.jointcommission.org).
- Develop intrahospital and agency safe transfer policies.

CHAIN OF COMMAND

The RN, including the new graduate nurse, is accountable to the charge nurse/nurse manager of the unit. The charge nurse is accountable to the nurse manager. The nurse manager is accountable to the chief nursing executive, such as the vice president for nursing. The chief nursing executive is accountable to the chief executive officer. The health care agency's chief executive officer is accountable to the board of directors. The board of directors is accountable to the community it serves and often to another larger health care agency, as well as to state nursing and medical licensing boards and accreditation agencies, for example, the American Osteopathic Association, Healthcare Facilities Accreditation Program (HFAP), and The Joint Commission. All are accountable for their actions to the patients and to the communities that they serve. See Figure 1-4.

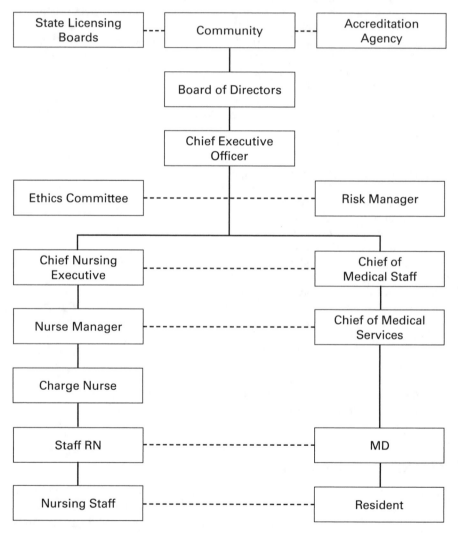

Figure 1-4 Organizational chain of command. (Delmar Cengage Learning.)

CASE STUDY 1-1

After a two-week orientation to the hospital and unit, a newly hired RN will start taking care of patients. The assigned preceptor and new RN are getting reports from the night nurse, who has added various adjectives when referring to NAP, including "Lazy Daisy" and "Sleepy Betty." Everyone laughs at the negative comments. Two months later, the new RN is giving report and refers to NAP in the same derogatory manner.

Why is the new RN referring to NAP in such a derogatory manner? How should the new RN refer to NAP? How could this incident have been prevented?

CRITICAL THINKING AND DECISION MAKING

Delegation is a must for the new nurse, as well as for the experienced nurse. Gladwell (2008) highlights the "10,000-Hour Rule." This rule claims that the key to success in any field is, to a large extent, a matter of practicing a specific task for a total of around 10,000 hours. Benner's (2001) work reminds us that nurses need information and the opportunity for skill building in delegation, especially at the start of their career. See Table 1-4.

The Pew Health Professions Commission identified that nurses must "demonstrate critical thinking, reflection, and problem-solving skills" in order to thrive as effective practitioners in the twenty-first century (Bellack & O'Neill, 2000). Paul (1992) defines **critical thinking** as "thinking about your thinking while you're thinking in order to make your thinking better" (p. 7). A critical thinker is able to examine decisions from all sides and take into account varying points of view. A critical thinker does not say, "We've always done it this way," and refuse to consider alternate ways. Rather, the critical thinker generates new ideas and alternatives when making decisions. The critical thinker asks "why?" questions about a situation in order to arrive at the best decision. Four basic skills—critical reading, critical listening, critical writing, and critical speaking—are necessary for the development of critical thinking skills. These skills are developed as part of the process of developing and using thinking for decision making. Ability in these four areas can be measured by the extent to which one uses the Universal Intellectual Standards listed in the left-hand column of Table 1-5. For example, a critical thinker works to be clear, precise, specific, accurate, and so on.

As you begin to apply critical thinking to nursing, use these Universal Intellectual Standards. Ask yourself whether the ideas are clear or unclear, precise or imprecise, specific or vague, accurate or inaccurate, and so forth.

TABLE 1-4

APPLICATION OF DELEGATION IN BENNER'S MODEL: NOVICE TO EXPERT

Benner's Model: Novice to Expert	Application to Delegation
Novice nurses are recognized as being task-oriented and focused on the rules. They tend to see nursing as a list of tasks to do rather than seeing the bigger picture of total patient care needed to meet patient care goals. Once novices have mastered most tasks required to perform their ascribed roles, they move on to the phase of advanced beginner.	The novice nurse is new to the direct patient care setting. The novice may have been educated in principles of delegation, but has not used them in the clinical setting. Novices are task-oriented, focused on perfecting their own skills, and are often still in orientation. Novices may begin to delegate tasks clearly outlined by the hospital. For instance, they may ask NAP to distribute drinking water to patients, but they often cannot decide what else to delegate. The novice tries to do all the tasks without help and may be slow to recognize the need to utilize NAP for successful patient care.
The advanced beginner is the nurse who can demonstrate marginally acceptable independent performance. This nurse still focuses on the rules but is more experienced. The advanced beginner still needs help identifying priorities.	This nurse is out of orientation and has worked for just a short while on the unit. The advanced beginner is able to perform most nursing tasks that are required for patient care. This nurse is becoming more comfortable delegating simple tasks to NAP, such as errands, assisting in positioning of patients, bathing, and taking vital signs. This nurse is often reluctant to delegate to any staff whose personality is resistant to his or her delegation. The advanced beginner nurse often needs to develop his or her organizational and time management skills and ability to manage a group of patients. This nurse's clinical skills, teamwork, and leadership skills still need development.
Competent nurses have been in their role for several years. These nurses have developed the ability to see their actions as part of the long-range	Several years in the same role allows nurses to develop the ability to see their actions as part of the long-range goals set for their

(continues)

Table 1-4 *(continued)*

goals set for their patients. They lack the speed of the proficient nurse, but they are able to manage most aspects of clinical care.

patients. These nurses delegate tasks to NAP so that the nurse is free to perform higher-level skills and make judgments. The competent nurse is able to assess the staff's abilities, communicate expectations effectively, and gather clinical information from staff members. This nurse is more comfortable delegating to staff even in the presence of personality conflicts. This nurse expects that all staff members meet the requirements of their job descriptions.

Proficient nurses characteristically perceive the whole situation rather than just seeing a series of tasks. They have often been on the job many years. They develop a plan of care and then guide the patient from Point A to Point B. They draw on their past experiences and know that in a typical situation, a patient must exhibit specific behaviors to meet specific goals. They realize that if those patient behaviors are not demonstrated within a certain time frame, then the plan of nursing care needs to be changed.

These nurses are often charge nurses developing plans of care for the whole unit. They see delegation and assignment of tasks as an important part of guiding patients from Point A to Point B. They are able to use past experiences with patients and staff to guide the delegation process.

Expert nurses are those nurses who intuitively know what is going on with their patients. Their expertise is so embedded in their practice that they have been heard to say, "There is something wrong with this patient. I'm not sure what is going on, but you had better come and evaluate the patient." Not heeding the observations derived from the intuitive sense of an expert nurse has resulted in patient deterioration and subsequent cardiac arrest. These expert nurses often seek advanced education.

These nurses are critical thinkers. They have knowledge about what is going on with their patients and what their patients' needs are. They can quickly assess what needs to be delegated and they evaluate the process of care continuously.

Adapted from *Novice to Expert: Excellence and Power in Clinical Nursing Practice*, by P. E. Benner, 2001. Upper Saddle River, NJ: Prentice Hall.

TABLE 1-5

THE SPECTRUM OF UNIVERSAL INTELLECTUAL STANDARDS

Clear _____	Unclear
Precise _____	Imprecise
Specific _____	Vague
Accurate _____	Inaccurate
Relevant _____	Irrelevant
Consistent _____	Inconsistent
Logical _____	Illogical
Deep _____	Superficial
Complete _____	Incomplete
Significant _____	Insignificant
Adequate _____	Inadequate
Fair _____	Unfair

Adapted from the Foundation for Critical Thinking, Dillon Beach, CA.
http://criticalthinking.org/

Nurses are expected to manage the care of a group of patients requiring specialized care to meet ultimate goals. It is not uncommon for nurses to assess, medicate, send a patient to surgery, and answer five phone calls within the first two hours of their shift. How does the nurse get everything done while providing quality care without becoming too overwhelmed? The use of critical thinking, decision making, and delegation is the answer.

Critical thinking is the use of thinking skills and abilities to make sound clinical judgments and safe decisions (Masters, 2009). Now, more than ever, nurses are required to think critically as technology and patient safety are combined with accountability and responsibility. The nurse must be able to think critically and utilize existing knowledge and skill to identify what should be done, what can be done and by whom, and what cannot be done. For example, a nurse was completing the following admitting orders: Take vital signs every four hours; obtain laboratory samples of CBC, PT, and PTT, blood cultures times two, and urinalysis; administer Ancef 1gram IVPB every eight hours; monitor Intake and Output; continue home meds; allow for a two-gram sodium diet; may have bathroom privileges; and insert IV lock. The nurse used critical thinking to determine that these orders were not to be completed in the order that they were written. The nurse first took a set of vital signs, then obtained the blood cultures and lab samples, and started the IV lock. Then the nurse administered Ancef. The other orders were then carried out. Assessment of a patient's vital signs and lab samples assures that he or she will receive the appropriate medications and treatments. Blood cultures must be drawn prior to administering an antibiotic.

DECISION-MAKING PROCESS AND DELEGATION

While decisions to delegate patient care are unique to different situations, the decision-making process can be applied to each situation. There are five steps in the decision-making process. Use of this five-step decision-making process will help the nurse make better decisions. See Table 1-6.

TABLE 1-6

DECISION-MAKING PROCESS

Five Steps of the Decision-Making Process
- Identify the need for a decision.
- Determine the goal or outcome.
- Identify alternatives or actions, and list the benefits and consequences of each.
- Choose an alternative.
- Evaluate the alternative chosen. Did you meet your goal?

From Decision making and critical thinking by S. Little-Stoetzel. In *Nursing leadership & management* (2nd ed.) (pp. 102–105) by P. Kelly, 2008. Clifton Park, NY: Delmar Cengage Learning.

CASE STUDY 1-2

Apply the decision-making process.
1. Identify the need for a decision.
   You are caring for Leona Glusak, who recently had a CVA. Her husband is worried about her and asks you if he can stay with her tonight. Mrs. Glusak was transferred from ICU two hours ago and is getting better.
2. Determine the goal or outcome.
   Your goal is to have both the patient and her husband maintain or improve their health. Mr. Glusak has told you that he has a heart condition himself. Staffing is good on the night shift.

(continues)

Case Study 1-2 *(continued)*

3. Identify alternatives or actions with benefits and consequences of each. The alternatives are:
   A. Let him stay. The benefits are that he won't be as worried. The consequences are that he may become exhausted over time.
   B. Talk with him and help him see the reasonableness of going home. The benefits are that he will get his rest. The consequences are that he may be thankful for the rest, especially if you take the time to talk with him. He could also become annoyed at being encouraged to go home. Or he may talk you into letting him stay the night.
   C. Send him home with no discussion. Enforce the unit's "No visitors at night" policy. The benefit is that this may help him rest. The consequences are that he may become angry and worried and not rest. He may also think the hospital staff is unkind or is hiding something.
4. Choose an alternative.
   B was chosen.
5. Evaluate the alternative chosen. Did you meet your goal?

EVIDENCE FROM THE LITERATURE

Citation: Bittner, N. P., & Gravlin, G. (2009). Critical thinking, delegation, and missed care in nursing practice. *Journal of Nursing Administration, 39*(3), 142–146.

Discussion: A qualitative, descriptive study examined how nurses use critical thinking to delegate nursing care. Prior to delegating, nurses considered the following: patient condition; competency, experience, and workload of nursing assistive personnel (NAP). Nurses expected NAP to report back to the RN significant findings and have higher level knowledge, including assessment and prioritizing skills. The relationship between the RN and NAP relating to communication, system support, and nursing leadership resulted in successful delegation. Nurses also reported frequent instances of missed or omitted routine care.

Implications for Practice: Ineffective delegation of basic nursing care can result in poor patient outcomes, potentially impacting quality measures, patient satisfaction, and reimbursement for the organization. Strategies to mitigate the consequence of missed care based on the findings is the challenge for all nurses.

REVIEW QUESTIONS

1. What types of information are often discussed with new nurse employees during hospital orientation? Select all that apply.
   ____ A. Nurse Practice Act
   ____ B. NAP job description
   ____ C. Hospital policy for delegation of duties
   ____ D. LPN/LVN job description

2. When a nurse asks another nurse to observe his or her group of patients while the first nurse is at lunch, and one patient falls out of bed, which nurse is responsible?
   A. The nurse originally assigned to the patient who went to lunch is responsible.
   B. The nurse who was observing the group of patients is responsible.
   C. Neither nurse is responsible.
   D. The action of both nurses will be reviewed.

3. After a patient's blood transfusion is completed, which health care personnel can obtain the vital signs? Select all that apply.
   ____ A. RN
   ____ B. LPN/LVN
   ____ C. NAP
   ____ D. New graduate nurse

4. A new graduate nurse is assigned a patient who is two days postoperative and has had a colostomy. The patient has an order to have a nasogastric tube inserted immediately. The new graduate has never inserted this type of tube in a patient. How should the new graduate nurse proceed in this situation?
   A. Delegate the task to NAP.
   B. Read over the procedure, and then insert the tube.
   C. Notify the health care provider of the new graduate's inexperience.
   D. Ask an experienced RN for assistance with the procedure.

5. The charge nurse working with an RN, an LPN, and a NAP is very busy with the group of patients on the unit. One patient's intravenous line has just infiltrated, a practitioner is on the phone waiting for a nurse's response, a patient wants to be discharged, and the NAP has just reported an elevated temperature on a new surgical patient. Who should be assigned to restart the intravenous line?
   A. LPN
   B. NAP
   C. RN
   D. Charge nurse

6. What knowledge of delegating patient care in a hospital setting is required to facilitate safe patient care?
   A. NAP is assigned patients to provide total patient care.
   B. NAP and RNs are to perform patient care when call lights are turned on.
   C. RNs are accountable for all patient care.
   D. LPN/LVNs are allowed to delegate patient care tasks to RNs.

7. A nurse interviewing for a job at a local hospital asked the recruiter to explain the roles of NAP. Which NAP role below should the nurse question?
   A. Passing water to patients
   B. Taking routine vital signs
   C. Completing a patient's list of belongings
   D. Notifying a family of the death of their loved one

8. Twenty-two patients are hospitalized on a locked psychiatric unit. Four of the patients are on suicide precautions. Two RNs and two NAP are assigned to the unit for the shift. The charge nurse calls the nursing supervisor and verbalizes the staff's concerns regarding inadequate staffing. What organizational accountability for delegation is referred to in this scenario?
   A. Provide adequate staffing with an appropriate staff mix
   B. Provide administrative support for supervisors and staff who delegate
   C. Provide documentation of routine maintenance for all patient care equipment
   D. Develop physical, mental, and verbal "No Abuse" polices to be followed by all professional and non-professional health care staff

9. NAP were each told by the charge nurse to take vital signs at 8:00 a.m. and 12:00 noon, turn patients who are on bed rest every two hours, and report their work completed to the RN caring for their patients. What is the rationale for NAP reporting to the RN that the tasks are completed?
   A. NAP are accountable both to the RN and the charge nurse.
   B. NAP are accountable only to the charge nurse since this is the nurse who delegated the tasks.
   C. NAP are accountable only to the RN caring for their patient.
   D. NAP are accountable to the patient.

10. The nurse asks a NAP who works on the nurse's unit and is also a nursing student if he/she wants to flush an IV site after the antibiotic infuses. The NAP enthusiastically answers "Yes." Is it okay for the NAP to flush the IV alone?
    A. No, because the NAP has not yet learned this skill in a clinical lab
    B. Yes, as long as the NAP has been taught how to flush an IV site

C. No, it is beyond the NAP's scope of practice

D. No, unless the patient agrees to have the NAP flush the IV

11. A new graduate nurse asks the charge nurse, "How do I know what I can and cannot delegate?" What is the best reply?

   A. "Delegation takes time and practice to learn what you can and cannot do."

   B. "If you follow the Five Rights of Delegation, you should be fine."

   C. "Every state has standards, laws, and guidelines for delegation to guide you."

   D. "You will not be delegating; only the charge nurse delegates, so there is nothing to worry about."

APPLY YOUR SKILLS

1. Read the article "Voluntary Overtime, Unsafe Nursing Practice, and the Quest for Institutional Accountability" by LaTonia D. Wright in the April/June 2007 *Journal of Nursing Administration's Healthcare, Law, Ethics and Regulation*. What has the author identified as the organizational accountability that impacts delegation of care?

2. Take an informal survey of NAP on the unit where you are doing your clinical practicum. Ask them what duties they have been given. Ask them whether there are any duties with which they are not comfortable. Discuss your findings.

3. Based on your observations of patient care delegation on your unit, which of the obstacles identified in Table 1-2 are present? Have you seen a lack of knowledge of job descriptions interfere with delegation? Have you seen a lack of confidence interfere with delegation? What else have you observed?

4. Identify a delegation problem that you have been considering. Using the decision-making grid at the bottom of this page, rate the alternative solutions to the problem that you have been considering on a scale of 1 to 3 on the elements of cost, quality, importance, and any other elements that are important to you.

   Did this exercise help you to clarify your thinking?

	Cost	Quality	Importance	Other
Alternative A				
Alternative B				
Alternative C				

5. At clinical, use a copy of the assignment sheet in Figure 1-2 to make assignments for a group of patients on your clinical unit. Identify who should fill out the assignment sheet. Who should be assigned what type of care and tasks for the group of patients?

EXPLORING THE WEB

1. Review the NCLEX test plan for information on the behaviors and content that will be tested. Search for "Test Plan" at www.ncsbn.org.
2. Visit www.ncsbn.org and review the job description of MA-C, the new addition to the NAP job description list. Find your state's definition of NAP and determine if MA-C are utilized.
3. Go to the ANA Web site, www.nursingworld.org, and type in "delegation," "supervision," and "authority" (terms discussed in this chapter) to review up-to-date position papers.
4. Check this list of favorite health care Web sites.

www.ahrq.gov	www.ngc.gov
www.ania.org	www.nih.gov
www.cdc.gov	www.nln.org
www.centerforamericannurses.org	www.nursingalliance.org
www.cms.hhs.gov	www.nursingcenter.com
www.cochrane.org	www.nursinglibrary.org
www.fda.gov	www.nursingworld.org
www.healthfinder.gov	www.osteopathic.org
www.healthgrades.com	www.pdr.net
www.jointcommission.org	www.psniwa.org
www.medlineplus.gov	www.rxlist.com
www.medscape.com	www.vh.org
www.ncsbn.org	

All accessed February 1, 2010

REFERENCES

American Association of Critical Care Nurses (AACN). (2004). AACN Delegation Handbook. Aliso Viejo, CA: Author.

American Nurses Association (ANA). (2005a). *Code of ethics for nurses with interpretive statements*. Washington, DC: American Nurses Publishing.

American Nurses Association (ANA). (2005b). *Principles for delegation*. Silver Spring, MD: American Nurses Association.

American Nurses Association (ANA) and National Council of State Boards of Nursing (NCSBN). (2006). *Joint statement on delegation.* Retrieved from www.ncsbn.org/Joint_statement.pdf

American Organization of Nurse Executives. (2003). *Healthy work environments, Vol. 2: Striving for excellence.* Retrieved September 1, 2008, from www.aone.org/aone/keyissues/hwe_excellence.html

Bellack, J. P., & O'Neill, E. H. (2000). Recreating nursing practice for a new century: Recommendations and implications of the Pew Health Professions Commission's final report. *Nursing and Health Care Perspectives, 21*(1), 14–21.

Benner, P. E. (2001). *From novice to expert: Excellence and power in clinical nursing practice.* Upper Saddle River, NJ: Prentice Hall.

Benner, P., Tanner, C. A., & Chesla, C. A. (1996). *Expertise in nursing practice: Caring clinical judgment and ethics.* New York, NY: Springer Publishing Company.

Bittner, N. P., & Gravlin, G. (2009). Critical thinking, delegation, and missed care in nursing practice. *Journal of Nursing Administration, 39*(3), 142–146.

Canadian Nurses Association. (2004). Promoting continuing competence for registered nurses. Ottawa, Canada: Author.

Center for American Nurses. (2008). *Registered nurse utilization of nursing assistive personnel: Statement for adoption.* Retrieved September 6, 2008, from www.centerforamericannurses.org/positions/finalassistivepersonnel.pdf

Cox, S. H. (1997, November). *Motivation and morale: Coin of the realm.* Symposium conducted at Nursing Management Congress. Dillon Beach, CA: Foundation for Critical Thinking.

Dillon Beach, CA: Foundation for Critical Thinking. http://criticalthinking.org

Gladwell, M. (2008). *Outliers.* Boston, MA: Little, Brown and Company.

Hansten, R. I., & Jackson, M. J. (2009). *Clinical delegation skills* (4th ed.). Sudbury, MA: Jones and Bartlett.

Hudspeth, R. (2007). Understanding delegation is a critical competency for nurses in the new millennium. *Nursing Administration Quarterly, 31*(2), 183–184.

Little-Stoetzel, S. (2008). Decision making and critical thinking. In P. Kelly (Ed.), *Nursing leadership & management* (2nd ed) (pp. 102–105). Clifton Park, NY: Delmar Cengage Learning.

Marthaler, M. (2009). Delegation. In D. Huber (Ed.), *Nursing leadership and management* (6th ed.) (p. 177). Missouri: Saunders.

National Council of State Boards of Nursing. (1995). *Delegation concepts and decision-making process.* Retrieved from www.ncsbn.org

Nightingale, F. (1859). *Notes on nursing: What is and what is not.* London, UK: Harrison & Sons.

Paul, R. (1992). *Critical thinking: What every person needs to survive in a rapidly changing world.* Santa Rosa, CA: Foundation of Critical Thinking.

SUGGESTED READINGS

International Council of Nurses. (2006). *International Council of Nurses Code of Ethics.* Geneva, Switzerland: International Council of Nurses.

Lanksbear, A., Sheldon, T., & Maynard, A. (2005). Nurse staffing and healthcare outcomes: A systematic review of the international research evidence. *Advances in Nursing Science, 28*(2), 163–174.

Mark, B. A., & Harless, D. W. (2007, Summer). Nurse staffing, mortality, and length of stay in for-profit and not-for-profit hospitals. *Inquiry, 44,* 167–186.

Masters, K. (2009). *Role development in professional nursing practice.* Sudbury, MA: Jones and Bartlett Publishers.

Ponte, P. R., Glazer, G., Dann, E., McCollum, K., Gross, A., Tyrrell, R., et al. (2007). The power of professional nursing practice: An essential element of patient and family centered care. *Online Journal of Issues in Nursing, 12.* Retrieved May 14, 2009, from http://nursingworld.org/ojin

Potter, P., & Grant, E. (2004). Understanding RN and unlicensed assistive personnel working relationships in designing care delivery strategies. *Journal of Nursing Administration, 34*(1), 19–25.

Tourigny, L., & Pulich, M. (2006). Delegating decision making in health care organizations. *The Health Care Manager, 25*(2), 101–113.

CHAPTER 2
NCSBN Delegation Decision-Making Tree and the Five Rights

Maureen T. Marthaler, Terry W. Miller, Richard J. Maloney,
Patsy Maloney, Patricia Kelly

> You have to be the change you want to see in the world.
>
> —Mahatma Gandhi

OBJECTIVES

Upon completion of this chapter, the reader should be able to:

1. Utilize the National Council of State Boards of Nursing (NCSBN) Decision-Making Tree.

2. List the Five Rights of Delegation.

3. Discuss the regulation of delegation.

4. Discuss sources of power.

5. Identify delegation responsibilities of health care team members.

6. Review delegation suggestions for registered nurses (RNs).

Stewart Biggos is a 10-year-old patient with diabetes mellitus. He is on bed rest, but wants to get out of bed and walk around. He has been dizzy at times since his admission.

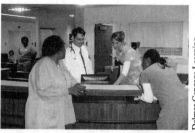

What tasks would you delegate to nursing assistive personnel (NAP)?

How would you retain responsibility and accountability for Stewart's care delivery?

The National Council of State Boards of Nursing (NCSBN) has developed a Delegation Decision-Making Tree for the nurse to use in delegating patient care. The Tree evaluates such elements as the competency of the nurse and nursing assistive personnel (NAP), as well as the stability of the patient in order to determine if patient care can be delegated.

This chapter will discuss this Tree, the role of state boards of nursing in delegation, delegation responsibilities of health care team members, the Five Rights of Delegation, sources of power, and other delegation suggestions for nurses.

THE NATIONAL COUNCIL OF STATE BOARDS OF NURSING DELEGATION DECISION-MAKING TREE

The steps of the Delegation Decision-Making Tree are as follows:
- Assessment of the patient, staff, and situational context and planning of the delegation based on patient needs and available resources
- Communication with the delegate to provide direction and opportunity for interaction during the completion of the delegated task, including any unique patient requirements and characteristics as well as clear expectations regarding what to do, what to report, and when to ask for assistance
- Surveillance, supervision, and monitoring of the delegation to assure compliance with standards of practice, policies, and procedures. This includes the level of supervision needed for the particular situation and the implementation of that supervision, including follow-up for problems or a changing situation.
- Evaluation and feedback to consider the effectiveness of the delegation, including any need to adjust the plan of care to achieve desired patient outcomes. See Figure 2-1.

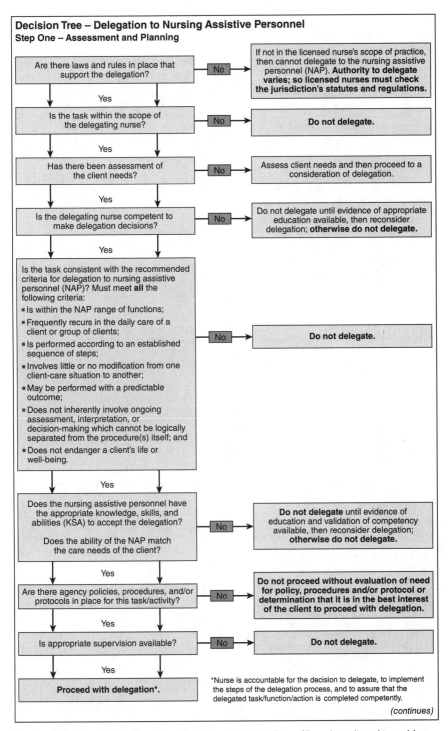

Figure 2-1 NCSBN Delegation Decision-Making Tree. (Reprinted and used by permission of the National Council of State Boards of Nursing, copyright 1997.)

Decision Tree – Delegation to Nursing Assistive Personnel *(continued)*
Step Two – Communication
Communication must be a two-way process.

The nurse:	*The nursing assistive personnel:*	*Documentation:*

▪ Assesses the assistant's understanding of:
 ▫ How the task is to be accomplished
 ▫ When and what information is to be reported, including:
  ▪ Expected observations to report and record
  ▪ Specific client concerns that would require prompt reporting.
▪ Individualizes for the nursing assistive personnel and client situation
▪ Addresses any unique client requirements, characteristics, and expectations
▪ Assesses the assistant's understanding of expectations, providing clarification if needed
▪ Communicates his or her willingness and availability to guide and support assistant
▪ Assures appropriate accountability by verifying that the receiving person accepts the delegation and accompanying responsibility.
	▪ Asks questions regarding the delegation and seeks clarification of expectations if needed
	▪ Informs the nurse if the assistant has not done a task/function/activity before, or has only done it infrequently
	▪ Asks for additional training or supervision
	▪ Affirms understanding of expectations
	▪ Determines the communication method between the nurse and the assistive personnel
	▪ Determines the communication and plan of action in emergency situations.
		Timely, complete, and accurate documentation of provided care
		▪ Facilitates communication with other members of the health care team
		▪ Records the nursing care provided.

Step Three – Surveillance and Supervision
The purpose of surveillance and monitoring is related to nurse's responsibility for client care within the context of a client population. The nurse supervises the delegation by monitoring the performance of the task or function and assures compliance with standards of practice, policies, and procedures. Frequency, level, and nature of monitoring vary with needs of client and experience of assistant.

The nurse considers the:	*The nurse determines:*	*The nurse is responsible for:*
▪ Client's health care status and stability of condition ▪ Predictability of responses and risks ▪ Setting where care occurs ▪ Availability of resources and support infrastructure ▪ Complexity of the task being performed.	▪ The frequency of onsite supervision and assessment based on: ▫ Needs of the client ▫ Complexity of the delegated function/task/activity ▫ Proximity of nurse's location.	▪ Timely intervening and follow-up on problems and concerns. Examples of the need for intervening include: ▫ Alertness to subtle signs and symptoms (which allows nurse and assistant to be proactive, before a client's condition deteriorates significantly) ▫ Awareness of assistant's difficulties in completing delegated activities ▫ Providing adequate follow-up to problems and/or changing situations, a critical aspect of delegation.

Step Four – Evaluation and Feedback
Evaluation is often the forgotten step in delegation.

In considering the effectiveness of delegation, the nurse addresses the following questions:
▪ Was the delegation successful?
 ▫ Was the task/function/activity performed correctly?
 ▫ Was the client's desired and/or expected outcome achieved?
 ▫ Was the outcome optimal, satisfactory, or unsatisfactory?
 ▫ Was communication timely and effective?
 ▫ What went well; what was challenging?
 ▫ Were there any problems or concerns; if so, how were they addressed?
▪ Is there a better way to meet the client need?
▪ Is there a need to adjust the overall plan of care, or should this approach be continued?
▪ Were there any "learning moments" for the assistant and/or the nurse?
▪ Was appropriate feedback provided to the assistant regarding the performance of the delegation?
▪ Was the assistant acknowledged for accomplishing the task/activity/function?

Figure 2-1 *(continued)*

THE FIVE RIGHTS OF DELEGATION

The NCSBN developed the Five Rights of Delegation in 1995. Eleven years later, in 2006, the American Nurses Association (ANA) and the NCSBN Joint Statement on Delegation clarified the Five Rights of Delegation as: The right task; Under the right circumstances; To the right person; With the right directions and communication; and Under the right supervision and evaluation. These Five Rights are used by the nurse who delegates patient care. See Table 2-1.

TABLE 2-1 *FIVE RIGHTS OF DELEGATION*	
The Right Task	• Has the organization established policies and standards consistent with the state nurse practice act; federal, state, and local regulations and guidelines for practice; nursing professional standards; and the ANA Code of Ethics (ANA, 2005)? • Can this task be delegated to any staff? • Are patient and community needs met?
Under the Right Circumstances	• Are the setting and available resources conducive to safe care? • Does staff understand how to do the task safely? • Does the job description, education, and competency of the RN, LPN/LVN, and NAP match the tasks? • Does staff do delegated tasks correctly? • Does staff have the resources, equipment, and supervision needed to work safely?
To the Right Person	• Is the right person delegating the right task to the right person to be performed on the right patient? • Is the patient stable with predictable outcomes? • Is it legally acceptable to delegate to this person? • Do personnel have documented knowledge, skill, and competency to perform the task?
With the Right Directions and Communication	• Does the RN communicate the task clearly with directions, specific steps of the task, limits, and expected outcomes? • Are times for feedback specified? • Is staff understanding of the task clarified? • Can staff say, "I don't know how to do this and I need help," without jeopardizing their job?

(continues)

Table 2-1 *(continued)*

Under the Right Supervision and Evaluation	• Is there appropriate monitoring, intervention, evaluation, and feedback as needed? • Does the RN answer staff questions and problem-solve as needed? • Does the staff report task completion and patient response to the RN? • Does the RN provide follow-up teaching and guidance to staff as appropriate? • Are problems, particularly any sentinel events, clarified or reported via the chain of command and as needed to the state board of nursing and accrediting agency?

Adapted from American Nurses Association and National Council of State Boards of Nursing, (2006), *Joint Statement on Delegation*. Retrieved December 1, 2009, from www.ncsbn.org

When an RN decides to delegate to others, he or she considers the needs and condition of the patient, potential harm, stability of the patient's condition, the task itself, the ability to predict outcomes, and knowledge of the staff's competencies. Principles for protecting the health, safety, and welfare of the public are also the basis for delegation. Figure 2-2 is an example of a critical-thinking grid that Seton Healthcare Network uses to assist its nurses to delegate.

REGULATION

The nursing profession determines what the definition of delegation is, as well as the nurse's role within the scope of nursing practice. The ANA and NCSBN define and guide the education, training, and utilization for not only the nursing profession but also any NAP. State Boards of Nursing define the legal parameters for RNs in their state nurse practice acts. Many state nurse practice acts specify nursing tasks that may be delegated as identified in Table 2-2.

Nurses can expect that the organization they work for will involve nurses in the development of policies related to delegating and assigning care. The organizational policies, procedures, and job descriptions should be congruent with the state nursing practice act. The organization is accountable for allocating resources for adequate staffing to allow the nurse to delegate appropriately. The organization is accountable for documenting

TABLE 2-2
DELEGATION EXAMPLES

Nursing Tasks That May *Not* Be Delegated
- Patient assessment (physical, psychological, and social assessment that requires professional nursing judgment, intervention, referral, or follow-up). Note that data collection without interpretation is not assessment.
- Planning of nursing care and evaluation of the patient's response to the care given
- Implementation of patient care that requires judgment
- Health teaching and health counseling other than reinforcement of what the RN has already taught
- Evaluation of the patient's response

Tasks That Are Most Commonly Delegated
- Non-invasive and non-sterile treatments
- Collecting, reporting, and documentation of data, such as
  - Vital signs, height, weight, intake and output
  - Ambulation, positioning, and turning
  - Transportation of the patient within the facility
  - Personal hygiene and elimination, including cleansing enemas
  - Feeding, cutting up of food, or placing of meal trays
  - Socialization activities
  - Activities of daily living

Nursing Tasks That May *Not* Be Routinely Delegated
Note that these may sometimes be delegated if the staff have received special credentialing, such as education and competency testing.
- Sterile procedures
- Invasive procedures, such as inserting tubes in a body cavity or instilling or inserting substances into an indwelling tube
- Care of broken skin other than minor abrasions or cuts generally classified as requiring only first-aid treatment
- Medication administration
- Transportation of the patient who requires constant cardiac monitoring within a facility
- Intravenous therapy

competencies for all staff providing direct patient care and for ensuring that the RN has access to competency information for personnel to whom the RN is delegating or assigning patient care (ANA and NCSBN, 2006). Implementing a system that ensures continued education of the staff to maintain competencies is an organizational responsibility as well.

BNE	TASK/PROCEDURE			PATIENT		UAP		RN
	Safety of Task	Absence of Problem-Solving	Interactions of RN to Patient	Stability of Patient for Task Per RN Assessment	Predict-ability of Patient's Response to Task	Validation of Competency	Experience	Availability
C A T E G O R I E S	High chance of risk; difficult to treat	Potential innovations that are not clearly defined	Require ongoing RN instruction throughout procedure	Unstable; probable fluctuation if task is done	Predictable negative response	No validation of competency	No experience with task or patient type	Not available
	0	0	0	0	0	0	0	0
	Moderate chance of risk; treatable over time	Options for innovations are clearly defined, but require a choice	Require intermittent interactions by RN throughout procedure	Currently stable; possible fluctuation if task is done	Response could be negative or positive	Validation of competency: *Discretionary Deleg.* Org. approved educ. program	Minimal experience with task and/or patient type	Available by phone or in person over time
	1	1	1	1	1	1	1	1

Figure 2-2 Seton Healthcare Network, RN Critical-Thinking Grid for Delegation to UAP (unlicensed assistive personnel). (Courtesy and used by permission of Joyce Batcheller, senior vice president, chief nursing officer, Seton Healthcare Network, Austin, Texas.)

(continues)

	TASK/PROCEDURE			PATIENT		UAP		RN
O **F**	Low chance of risk; easily treatable, temporary	Problem-solving has clearly defined option identified in procedure/education	RN interactions completed before and/or after procedure	Stable; fluctuations unlikely if task is done	Minimal chance of negative response	Validation of competency; *Discretionary Deleg.* Org. approved educ. Program	Recent or frequent experience with task and/or patient type	Available; easy to find
	2	2	2	2	2	2	2	2
T **A** **S** **K** **S**	Minimal or no chance of risk; no treatment needed	No innovations needed	No RN interactions needed	Consistently stable; no expected fluctuations if task is done	Predictable favorable response	*Most Commonly Deleg. Tasks* Competency validation per delegating RN	Experience with specific task and patient	Immediately available
	3	3	3	3	3	3	3	3

SCALE
0 = Not Met
1 = Marginally Met
2 = Adequately Met
3 = Ideally Met

Figure 2-2 *(continued)*

The final decision for delegation is based upon the RN's professional judgment. (BNE 218.10.6)

Guidelines for Decision Making

☐ If a "0" is selected for any of the criterion in any of the categories (RN, UAP, PATIENT, or TASK), it is recommended that the task *not* be delegated.

☐ If a "1" is selected in the RN or UAP categories, it is recommended that all criterion in the PATIENT and "TASK" categories be a "2" or "3".

☐ If a "1" is selected for any of the PATIENT or TASK categories, it is recommended that all criterion in the RN and UAP category be a "2" or "3".

☐ If a "2" or "3" is selected for each of the criterion in the PATIENT, TASK, RN, or UAP categories, the task may be delegated.

☐ Category "3" represents the ideal criterion for delegation.

EVIDENCE FROM THE LITERATURE

Citation: Nursing and Midwifery Council. (2008, May). Advice on delegation for registered nurses and midwives. Retrieved December 1, 2009, from www.nmc-uk.org

Discussion: This article provides advice on delegation to nurses and midwives in the United Kingdom (UK). Nurses in the United States can also use this advice. The Nursing and Midwifery Council is the United Kingdom's regulatory body organization for nursing and midwifery. The primary purpose of the Council is to protect the public. This role is similar to the role of the state boards of nursing in the United States. Non-regulated personnel is the term in the UK for NAP. The term *registrant* is the UK term for *nurse*.

When a nurse or midwife has authority to delegate tasks to another, he or she will retain responsibility and accountability for that delegation. A nurse or midwife may only delegate an aspect of care to a person deemed competent to perform the task. The nurse or midwife should be sure that the person to whom care has been delegated fully understands the nature of the delegated task and what is required. Where another person, such as an employer, has the authority to delegate an aspect of care, the employer becomes accountable for that delegation. The nurse or midwife will, however, continue to carry the responsibility to intervene if he or she feels that the proposed delegation is inappropriate or unsafe. The decision whether or not to delegate an aspect of care and to transfer and/or to rescind delegation is the primary responsibility of the nurse or midwife and is based on his or her professional judgment.

Nurses or midwives have the right to refuse to delegate if they believe that it would be unsafe to do so or if they are unable to provide or ensure adequate supervision. Those delegating care and those assuming delegated duties should do so in accordance with robust local employment practice in order to protect the public and support safe practice.

Implications for practice: The decision to delegate is made either by the nurse, midwife, or by the employer, and it is this decision maker who is accountable for the decision. Health care can sometimes be unpredictable. It is important that the person to whom an aspect of care is being delegated understands his or her limitations. He or she must know when not to proceed should circumstances affecting the task change. No one should feel pressured into either delegating or accepting a delegated task. When pressure is felt, advice should be sought, as appropriate, from either the nurse or the midwife's professional manager.

KNOWLEDGE AND SKILLS OF DELEGATION

Delegation is not a skill that is simply learned in a classroom. Delegation requires discussion of knowledge and skills related to delegation and clinical mentorship, or practice in responsibilities related to that delegation. This discussion of knowledge and skills related to delegation should be provided by undergraduate nursing education, as well as by the organization that is orienting RNs and NAP. Job descriptions must be clarified. Lack of clear job descriptions for the RN and NAP results in frustration and resistance to delegation. NAP jobs that have a certification requirement promote confidence in the nurse to delegate. For example, the NCSBN *Medication Assistant-Certified (MA-C) Model Curriculum* (2007) explicitly defines the role of the MA-C. NAP who have earned this title can administer medications under the supervision of a nurse in accordance with the state nurse practice act. Other NAP positions are not always this clear. The RN who works with NAP must work to develop clear communication regarding all standards for safe patient care.

When a nurse gives a task to another nurse, they share the common bond of knowing their job description and the nurse practice act. The crash cart can be assigned to another nurse to be checked. The nurse assigning the task is familiar with the task and the nurse's ability to check the crash cart.

POWER

Nurses use power when delegating patient care to others. Most researchers agree that sources of power and authority for nurses are diverse and vary from one situation to another. Articles and textbooks about nursing administration, educational leadership, and classical organizational management include references to the work of Hersey, Blanchard, and Natemeyer (1979), which is an expansion of the power typology originally developed by French and Raven in 1959. This power typology helps nurses understand how different people perceive power and subsequently relate and delegate to others in the work setting to achieve patient care goals (Miller, Maloney, & Maloney, 2008). Power is described as having a basis in expertise, legitimacy, reference (charisma), reward, coercion, or connection. Generally speaking, nurses exert influence derived from one power source or a combination of power sources. See Table 2-3.

The way that power is used to delegate or accomplish a goal often determines its desirability and how others perceive it. Effective nurses use sources of power, as appropriate, when delegating care. They

TABLE 2-3
SOURCES OF POWER

Sources of Power	How Power Works
Expert Power (Fisher & Koch, 1996)	Expert power comes from the knowledge and skills that nurses possess. The greater any nurse's proficiency in performing his or her role, the greater the nurse's expert power. This power should be acknowledged by others to be most effective.
Legitimate Power (Fisher & Koch, 1996)	Legitimate power is derived from the position a nurse holds in a group, and it indicates the nurse's degree of authority. Legitimate power is based on such factors as licensure, academic degrees, certification, experience in the role, and title/position in the institution.
Referent (Charisma) Power (Fisher & Koch, 1996)	Referent power is derived from the admiration, trust, and respect that people feel toward an individual, group, or organization. The referent person has the ability to inspire confidence. In any situation, strong referent leaders are considered to be charismatic and people of great vision, which may or may not be the reality.
Reward or Coercion Power (Miller, 2008)	The ability to reward or punish others, as well as the power to create fear in others to influence them to change their behavior, is commonly termed reward power or coercive power.
Connection Power (Miller, 2003)	Both personal and professional relationships are part of a nurse's connections. People who are strongly connected to others, both personally and professionally, have enhanced resources and enhanced capacity for learning and sharing information. They have a broader overall sphere of influence. Teamwork, collaboration, networking, and mentoring are some of the ways that a nurse can become more connected and therefore more powerful.
Information Power (Miller, 2003)	Information power is power based on the information that any person can provide to the group. Authoritarian leaders attempt to control information. Charismatic leaders provide information that is seductive for many people. Information leaders provide a sense of stability with the use and synthesis of information. Some people believe the greatest power may be in information—if one knows how to obtain it and what to do with it.

(continues)

Table 2-3 *(continued)*

Subordinate Power (DuBrin, 2000)	Subordinate power is any type of power that employees can exert upward in their organization based on legal and justice considerations. When subordinates perceive an order as being outside the limits of legitimate authority, they have the power to rebel.

Adapted from Power, by T. Miller, R. Maloney, and P. Maloney. In *Nursing leadership & management* (2nd ed.) (pp. 170–173), by P. Kelly (Ed.), Clifton Park, NY: Delmar Cengage Learning.

combine referent (charismatic) power and expert power from a legitimate power base, adding carefully measured portions of reward and connection power and little or preferably no coercive power. These nurses gather and use information in new and creative ways. They understand that power should be a means to accomplish a goal instead of a goal in itself. Understanding and using these sources of power assists the nurse when delegating care.

RESPONSIBILITIES OF HEALTH CARE TEAM MEMBERS

The consequences and likely effects must be considered when delegating patient care. The AACN (2004) suggests assessment of five factors that must occur before deciding to delegate:

1. *Potential for Harm:* Determine if there is a risk for the patient in the activity delegated.
2. *Complexity of the Task:* Delegate simple tasks. These tasks often require psychomotor skills with little assessment or judgment proficiency.
3. *Amount of Problem Solving and Innovation Required:* Do not delegate simple tasks that require a creative approach, adaptation, or special attention to complete.
4. *Unpredictability of Outcome:* Avoid delegating tasks in which the outcome is not clear, causing volatility for the patient.
5. *Level of Patient Interaction:* Value time spent with the patient and the patient's family to develop trust, and so on.

Attention to these five factors will improve patient safety associated with delegation. A new graduate nurse may feel overwhelmed in his or her first nursing position by the responsibility of patient care, especially if patient needs are urgent. New nurses may quickly realize that if they do not delegate some of the patient's care, it will not be completed in a timely and effective manner. Other staff can assist new nurses by helping them develop their roles and teaching them how to delegate. Other staff can also help by introducing department staff and explaining their roles to the new nurses. Note that nurses can never delegate any part of the nursing process that requires specialized knowledge, judgment, and skill that only professional nurses are educated and licensed to do. Tasks that are appropriate to delegate often fall under the nursing process step of implementation and include measuring vital signs, bathing, and assisting with activities of daily living, etc.

Nurse Manager Responsibility

A nurse manager is an individual who coordinates actions and allocates resources in a unit or department to achieve organizational goals. A nurse manager has learned how to delegate to NAP and follows the Five Rights of Delegation.

The nurse manager also helps develop staff members' ability to delegate. Guidance in this area is necessary because new graduates, wanting to be regarded favorably, often try to do everything themselves and do not ask for assistance. Nursing orientation will cover staff job descriptions, competency, chain-of-command guidelines, and other organizational resources for the new nurse. Delegation is a skill that will require much guidance and practice.

Registered Nurse Responsibility

Many nurses are reluctant to delegate. This is reflected in anecdotal accounts from nursing students and practicing nurses. There are many contributing factors, e.g., not having had educational opportunities to learn how to work with others effectively, not knowing the skill level and abilities of NAP, the fast work pace, and the rapid turnover of patients. At the same time, there has been an increase in the amount and complexity of nursing tasks performed by assistive personnel. Nurses increasingly need the support of NAP.

The registered nurse (RN) is responsible and accountable for the provision of nursing care. Although NAP may measure vital signs, intake and output, and other patient status indicators, it is the RN who analyzes this data for comprehensive assessment, nursing diagnosis, implementation, and evaluation of the plan of care. The RN also remains responsible for the patient outcome.

NEW GRADUATE REGISTERED NURSE RESPONSIBILITY

Delegation skills are developed over time. Nursing employers need to recognize that a newly licensed nurse is a novice who is still acquiring foundational knowledge and skills. In addition, many nurses lack the knowledge, skill, and confidence to delegate effectively, so ongoing opportunities to use the Delegation Decision-Making Tree and apply the principles of delegation are an essential part of employment orientation and staff development.

New graduate RNs need to focus on the duties for which they are directly responsible. What duties can they delegate and to what extent? What do NAP do? What do licensed practical nurses/licensed vocational nurses (LPN/LVNs) do? The state nurse practice act and the job description of each of these staff will help clarify the responsibilities of each staff member.

LICENSED PRACTICAL/VOCATIONAL NURSE RESPONSIBILITY

LPN/LVN caregivers who have undergone a standardized training and competency evaluation are able to perform various duties. LPN/LVNs are held to a high standard of care and are responsible for their actions. LPN/LVNs usually care for stable patients with predictable outcomes, although they may help RNs care for seriously ill patients in the ICU. Common LPN/LVN duties include the duties of the NAP, as well as reinforcing teaching from a standard care plan and updating initial assessments. In many states, when LPN/LVNs have documented competency, their required duties may also include maintaining intravenous lines, administering blood transfusions, maintaining hyperalimentation lines, administering IV push and piggyback medications, and inserting nasopharyngeal or oropharyngeal feeding tubes, and so on. The LPN/LVN works under the direction of the RN. Their roles must be in agreement with the state nurse practice act and should be reflected in policies, job descriptions, methods of assigning duties, and competency documentation, no matter what the setting. See a sample scope of practice for licensed vocational nurses in Texas at www.bon.state.tx.us. Click on "Nursing Practice," then "Scope of Practice."

The RN must be aware of the job description, skills, and educational background of the LPN/LVN prior to delegation of duties. Note that the RN is still primarily responsible and accountable for overall patient assessment, nursing diagnosis, planning, implementation, and evaluation of the quality of care delegated to the LPN/LVN. See Figure 2-3.

Elements to Consider

- Federal, state, and local regulations and guide-lines for practice, in-cluding the state nurse practice act
- Nursing professional standards
- Organizational policy, procedure, and standards

- Job description of Registered Nurse, Licen-sed Practical Nurse/ Licensed Vocational Nurse, Nursing Assistive Personnel
- Five Rights of Delegation

- Knowledge and skill of personnel
- Documented personnel competency, strengths, and weaknesses (select the right person for the right job)
- ANA Principles of Dele-gation, i.e., overarching principles, nurse-related principles, and organizational-related principles

↓

RN is accountable for application of the nursing process:
- Assessment and nursing judgment*
- Nursing diagnosis
- Planning care
- Implementation and teaching
RN delegates as appropriate.
RN retains accountability.
Note that LPN/LVNs and NAP are also responsible for their actions.**

↓

RNs	**LPN/LVNs**	**NAP**
RNs assess, plan care, monitor, and evaluate all patients, especially com-plex, unstable patients with unpredictable outcomes.	LPN/LVNs care for stable patients with predictable outcomes. They work un-der the direction of the RN and are responsible for their actions within their scope of practice.	UAP assist the RNs and the LPN/LVNs and give technical care to stable patients with predictable outcomes and minimal potential for risk. They work under the direction of an RN and are respon-sible for their actions.
Administer medications, including IV Push and IVPBs.	Gather patient data.	Assist with activities of daily living.
Start and maintain IVs and blood transfusions.	Implement patient care.	
	Maintain infection control.	
	Provide teaching from standard teaching plan.	

(continues)

Figure 2-3 Considerations in delegation. (Delmar Cengage Learning.)

RNs	LPN/LVNs	NAP
Perform sterile or specialized procedures, i.e., Foley catheter and nasogastric tube insertion, tracheostomy care, suture removal, and so on.	Depending on the state and with documented competency, may do the following:**	Bathe, groom, and dress.
	• Administer medications.	Assist with toileting and bed making.
Educate patient and family.	• Perform sterile or specialized procedures, for example, Foley catheter and nasogastric tube insertion, tracheostomy care, suture removal, and so on.	Ambulate, position, and transport.
Maintain infection control.		Feed and socialize with patient.
Administer cardiopulmonary resuscitation.		Measure intake & output (I&O).
Interpret and report laboratory findings.	• Perform blood glucose monitoring.	Document care.
Triage patients.	• Administer CPR.	Weigh patient.
Prevent nurse-sensitive patient outcomes, for example, cardiac arrest, pneumonia, and so on.	• Perform venipuncture and insert peripheral IVs, change IV bags for patients receiving IV therapy, and so on.	Maintain infection control.
Monitor patient outcomes.		Depending on the state and with documented competency, may do the following:**
		• Perform blood glucose monitoring.
		• Collect specimens.
		• Administer CPR.
		• Take vital signs.
		• Perform 12-lead EKGs.
		• Perform venipuncture for blood tests.

Evaluation
RN uses judgment and is responsible for evaluation of all patient care.

*Nursing judgment is the process by which nurses come to understand the problems, issues, and concerns of patients, to attend to salient information, and respond to patient problems in concerned and involved ways. Judgment includes both conscious decision making and intuitive response (Benner, Tanner, & Chesla, 1996).

**Some variation from state to state and health care agency.

Figure 2-3 *(continued)*

KEEP YOUR PATIENTS SAFE 2-1

Identify a group of four patients on the unit where you have your clinical experience. Note the RNs, LPN/LVNs, and NAP on the unit. Practice delegation decision making using the Five Rights of Delegation and the NCSBN Delegation Decision-Making Tree with this group of patients and staff. How did it go? What issues did you have to work out? Would you make the same delegation decision again?

NURSING ASSISTIVE PERSONNEL RESPONSIBILITY

The increased numbers of NAP in acute care settings pose a degree of risk to the patient. The House of Representatives Patient Safety Act of 1996 assists in the campaign for safe staffing levels using an appropriate skill mix for patient outcomes. The Act assures that every patient is assigned an RN. According to the Act, NAP may perform duties such as bathing, feeding, toileting, and ambulating patients. NAP should also report information related to these activities. The RN will delegate to the NAP and is responsible and accountable for those delegated tasks. According to the ANA (2007), the RN must utilize the right and obligation to know that the NAP has appropriate training, orientation, and documented competencies. The RN can then reasonably expect that the NAP will function in a safe and effective manner. Of course, the RN remains responsible for ongoing patient safety.

Using NAP in acute care settings frees RNs from non-nursing duties and allows RNs time to complete assessments of patients and record their responses to treatments. It is less expensive to have NAP perform non-nursing duties than to have nurses perform them. NAP can deliver supportive care. They cannot practice nursing or provide total patient care. Inappropriate use of NAP in performing functions outside their scope of practice is a violation of the state nursing practice act and is a threat to patient safety. The RN must monitor patient care and patient outcomes when tasks are delegated to NAP. The RN must be aware of the job description, skills, educational background, and competency of the NAP prior to the delegation of duties.

Note that the Code for Federal Regulations 42 CFR § 483.156 requires that every state, as well as the District of Columbia, maintain a registry of all nurse's aides who work in long-term facilities that participate in Medicaid and Medicare. This is just a list of NAP. The registry does not include a job description or any standards of practice for the NAP. Additionally, a standard of practice across all states has not kept up with the needs of the residents of long-term care facilities. The lack of uniformity of job descriptions and required training even at the federal level has allowed the NAP role to be ambiguous.

REAL WORLD INTERVIEW

I have witnessed charge nurses delegating to make their workload easier to an extent far beyond what they should. Charge nurses have many duties and responsibilities. I have also observed charge nurses as well as other nurses delegating duties to staff that were not within their scope of practice. I have seen charge nurses delegate duties as a way of "picking" on someone, for example, by giving them the "worst" task. I have observed charge nurses failing to carry out their duties correctly or efficiently. For example, some charge nurses who are assigned to check the emergency supplies or crash carts do not really do this thoroughly or at all. Another example is the charge nurse who is not following up with or checking on the other staff nurses during the shift, or helping them with any problems they may have encountered.

My suggestions for accurate and fair delegation are, first of all, to assure that the charge nurse knows his or her responsibilities. Moreover, charge nurses as well as other staff nurses must be aware of the scope of practice for all other health care providers. Perhaps having an annual review or competency assessment for charge nurses would be helpful to fulfill this requirement. It is important for other staff members to know and utilize the chain of command, especially if they are constantly witnessing or experiencing incorrect delegation. Charge nurses must possess many qualities, such as honesty, patience, fairness, reliability, and knowledge of what is expected of them as well as of their fellow nurses. This is essential when providing patient-centered care.

Amy Pantaleo, RN, BSN
Munster, Indiana

KEEP YOUR PATIENTS SAFE 2-2

Identify which members of the health care team may perform each of the following nursing activities.

Nursing Activity	RN	LPN/LVN	NAP
Administer blood to a patient.			
Assess a patient going to surgery.			
Develop a teaching plan for a patient newly diagnosed with diabetes.			
Measure a patient's intake and output.			

(continues)

Keep Your Patients Safe 2-2 *(continued)*

Nursing Activity	RN	LPN/LVN	NAP
Give a bath to an immobilized patient.			
Perform a dressing change on a patient.			
Give patient report when transferring a patient from the ICU to a step-down unit.			
Administer insulin.			
Evaluate a patient's DNR status.			
Give an oral medication.			
Assist a patient with ambulation.			
Give an IM pain medication.			

KEEP YOUR PATIENTS SAFE 2-3

Note the following selected list of cultural values:

Mainstream American Values	Other Cultural Values
Make your own luck.	Fate and luck determine our life.
Like change.	Like tradition.
Arrive on time.	Frequently arrive late.
Value the individual.	Value the group.
Value competition.	Value cooperation.
Set goals for the future.	Enjoy life and just let it happen.
Value directness.	Value being subtle.
Believe that all people have a fairly equal chance to achieve status.	Believe that some people will always have higher status.

Which of these values do you hold? Which do members of your staff hold? What can you do to improve communication around these values and improve your working relationships?

DELEGATION SUGGESTIONS FOR RNS

RNs concerned with appropriate delegation may find it helpful to use the delegation suggestions in Tables 2-4 and 2-5.

TABLE 2-4
DELEGATION SUGGESTIONS FOR THE RN

- Consider prior to delegating:
  - Who has the time to complete the delegated task?
  - Who is the best person for the task?
  - What is the urgency of the task?
  - Are there any deadlines?
  - Which staff need to develop their skills?
  - Which staff would enjoy the task?
- Be clear about the qualifications of the delegate, such as education, experience, and competency. Require documentation or demonstration of current competence by the delegate for each task. Clarify patient care concerns or delegation problems. Click on ANA position statements at www.nursingworld.org and your state board of nursing, as necessary.
- Speak to your delegates as you would like to be spoken to. There is no need to apologize for your delegation. Remember, you are carrying out your professional responsibility.
- Communicate the patient's name, room number, and duty to be performed. Identify the time frame for completion. Discuss any changes from the usual procedures that might be needed to meet special patient needs and any potential patient abnormalities that should be reported to the RN. The expectations for personnel before, during, and after duty performance should be stated in a clear, pleasant, direct, and concise manner.
- Identify the expected patient outcome and the limits of the delegate's authority.
- Verify the delegate's understanding of delegated tasks and have the delegate repeat instructions, as needed. Verify that the delegate accepts responsibility and accountability for carrying out the task correctly. Require frequent mini-reports about patients from staff.
- Avoid removing duties once assigned. This should be considered only when the duty is above the level of the personnel, as when the patient's care is in jeopardy because the patient's status has changed.
- Monitor task completion according to standards. Make frequent walking rounds to assess patient outcomes.
- Accept minor variations in the style in which the duties are performed. Individual styles are acceptable if the standards are met and good outcomes are achieved.
- Try to meet staff needs for learning opportunities. Consider any health problems and work preferences of the staff as long as they don't interfere with meeting patient needs.

(continues)

Table 2-4 *(continued)*

- If a delegate doesn't meet the standards, talk with him or her to identify the problem. If this is not successful, inform the delegate that you will be discussing the problem with your supervisor. Document your concerns, as appropriate. Follow up with your supervisor according to your organization's policy.
- Treat others as you wish to be treated.
- Honor the culture of patients and staff.
- Take time to get to know your co-workers.
- Welcome new staff members.
- Delegate tasks to staff members who want to learn and are concerned about the patient's best interests.
- Communicate to the NAP, in a written or verbal format, the patient's name, room number, disease process, allergies, precautions, restraints, family concerns, and any other pertinent information.
- Delegate patient tasks and communicate expected patient outcomes, time line, frequency, limitations, and any other expectations the nurse may have.
- Assure the NAP that you are available to answer questions and provide assistance if needed.
- Help when you can. You may not always be able to help, but when you do help with tasks to be completed by the NAP, it is always worth 100 future favors.
- Prior to delegating to a NAP whom you are not familiar with, consider:
  ○ What are the NAP's qualifications? Where are the qualifications documented?
  ○ Has this task been delegated to any NAP before?
  ○ Has this task been delegated to this NAP before?
  ○ If the task has been delegated, what was the outcome? Was the task completed on time, accurately, without difficulty, and with appropriate frequency?
- Check the ANA position statements; state board of nursing nurse practice act, rules, and regulations; and your organization's policy and procedures.
- Avoid high-risk delegation. Patients will be at risk if you delegate a task that should be performed only by an RN according to law, organizational policies and procedures, or professional standards of nursing practice; if the delegated task could involve substantial risk or harm to a patient; if you knowingly delegate a task to a person who has not had the appropriate training or orientation; or if you fail to adequately supervise the delegated activities and do not evaluate the delegated action by reassessing the patient.

TABLE 2-5
DELEGATION CHECKLIST

Question	Yes	No
Do you recognize that you retain ultimate responsibility for the outcome of delegated assignments?	_____	_____
Do you spend most of your time completing tasks that require an RN?	_____	_____
Do you trust the ability of your staff to complete job assignments successfully?	_____	_____
Do you allow staff sufficient time to solve their own problems before interceding with advice?	_____	_____
Do you clearly outline expected outcomes and hold your staff accountable for achieving these outcomes?	_____	_____
Do you support your staff with an appropriate level of feedback and follow-up?	_____	_____
Do you use delegation as a way to help staff develop new skills and provide challenging work assignments?	_____	_____
Does your staff know what you expect of them?	_____	_____
Do you take the time to carefully select the right person for the right job?	_____	_____
Do you feel comfortable sharing control with your staff as appropriate?	_____	_____
Do you clearly identify all aspects of an assignment to staff when you delegate?	_____	_____
Do you assign tasks to the lowest level of staff capable of completing them successfully?	_____	_____
Do you support your staff, even when they are learning?	_____	_____
Do you allow your staff reasonable freedom to achieve outcomes?	_____	_____

Compiled with information from Harvard ManageMentor® Delegating Tools (2004). *Delegation skills checklist.* Boston, MA: Harvard Business School Publishing.

CASE STUDY 2-1

It is one hour prior to the end of a shift. The nurse on the telemetry floor with four patients asks the NAP for a list of the patients' intake and output (I&O) totals. The NAP stumbles for words, and the nurse impatiently says, "Forget it, I will just get them myself." The nurse walks away mumbling, "lazy, so darn lazy." The NAP smiles at one of the other NAP and says, "It works every time."

What could the nurse have done to better utilize the NAP in obtaining the I&O totals? When a nurse assumes the NAP will not complete a task and completes it himself or herself, what is likely to happen with future delegations to the NAP?

Choose a group of patients from the List of Patient Descriptions in the front of this book. You are the nurse working with an LPN/LVN and a NAP. Apply the four steps of the Delegation Decision-Making Tree in Figure 2-1. Decide what you can safely delegate to the LPN/LVN and NAP. Also, you may want to refer to Figure 2-3 as you decide.

REVIEW QUESTIONS

1. Which health care team members can reinforce patient teaching on how to use an incentive spirometer prior to discharge? Select all that apply.
   A. Respiratory therapist
   B. Licensed practical nurse
   C. Nursing assistive personnel
   D. Registered nurse

2. As a traveling nurse going from one hospital to another and from state to state, it can be difficult to identify the health care team members' roles. What information does the nurse need in regard to working with NAP? Select all that apply.
   A. Licensure
   B. Orientation received
   C. Training received
   D. Competencies documented

3. When a nurse considers delegating to a NAP, what Five Rights should be utilized?
   A. Right task, right circumstance, right person, right direction/communication, right supervision
   B. Right room, right time, right person, right documentation, right nurse

    C. Right patient, right chart, right doctor, right results, right information

    D. Right person, right patient, right task, right time frame, right side

4. A nurse has become incredibly busy with discharging two patients and is expecting a newly admitted patient any second. The following list of tasks needs to be completed right away. Which task can the nurse delegate to NAP?

    A. Provide tracheostomy care.

    B. Transport a patient on a cardiac monitor to X-ray.

    C. Remove sutures from an incision and drainage (I&D) of the left wrist.

    D. Sit with a patient who was recently diagnosed with Crohn's disease who is crying.

5. The staff working on a unit includes four RNs, two LPNs, and a NAP for 25 medical patients. What assignment is most appropriate for the LPN?

    A. Pass medications to a group of patients.

    B. Take a history on a newly admitted patient.

    C. Pass water to all of the patients on the unit.

    D. Obtain a urine sample from a patient's Foley catheter.

6. What is the most appropriate task for the RN to delegate to the NAP?

    A. Reset the IV pump until the nurse arrives.

    B. Notify the family of a patient who has died.

    C. Reinforce teaching for a patient who has an above-the-knee amputation (AKA).

    D. Administer a soapsuds enema to a patient.

7. An LPN is assigned to pass medications to seven patients. Several hours after the LPN was to finish passing the medications, one of the patients complained to the RN that he had not received his medication. How should the nurse handle this situation initially?

    A. Discuss the patient's complaint with the LPN.

    B. Ask all of the patients if they have received their medications.

    C. Disregard the patient's complaint and give him the medication.

    D. Follow the LPN during the next medication administration to verify that all medications are administered.

8. Who is legally responsible for the nursing care provided to patients?

    A. Nurse manager

    B. RN assigned to the patient

    C. Person providing care at the time

    D. Physician

9. A nurse delegated the turning of a particular patient to the NAP. After an hour had passed, the nurse asked the NAP if the patient had been turned. The NAP replied "No." What should the nurse have done initially to ensure that the task was completed in a timely fashion?
   A. Explained the procedure to the NAP
   B. Assisted the NAP in turning the patient
   C. Delegated this task to another staff member
   D. Informed the NAP of the time frame in which the task was to be completed

10. When the shift begins, what should be delegated to the NAP to be completed immediately?
   A. Turn off the IV pump alarm that is beeping.
   B. Pass fresh water to all of the patients.
   C. Take a set of vital signs on all of the patients.
   D. Assess a patient's pedal pulses following the previous day's femoral popliteal graft.

11. The NAP reports to the nurse that a patient is complaining of shortness of breath (SOB). Which task can the nurse delegate to the NAP?
   A. Listen to the patient's lungs.
   B. Position the patient in a high Fowler's position.
   C. Document the condition of the patient since the NAP is the person reporting it.
   D. Notify the respiratory therapist that the patient needs a breathing treatment.

12. The nurse activated an emergency code blue for a patient who had a respiratory arrest. The first person to arrive is a new NAP. What should the nurse delegate to the NAP to do first?
   A. Assist in cardiopulmonary resuscitation.
   B. Help the patient in the next bed leave the room.
   C. Call the family and notify them of the patient's condition.
   D. Start moving the bed of the patient who has arrested to the intensive care unit.

APPLY YOUR SKILLS

1. You just admitted a new patient. You are trying to decide whether to delegate his care to NAP Jill or to NAP Penny. Use the Decision-Making Grid in Table 2-6 to decide.

TABLE 2-6				
DECISION-MAKING GRID				
	Certified?	Easy to work with?	Does their fair share?	Other concerns?
Jill				
Penny				

2. It is not uncommon for nursing students to work in the hospital as NAP. Have you observed any skills delegated to students that are inappropriate for NAP to perform?

3. A 45-year-old male is admitted to the unit with a tentative diagnosis of liver tumor. He has been experiencing increasing fatigue, anorexia, and a steady weight loss of 20 pounds over the last few months. He is currently 6'2" and weighs 212 pounds. He has moderate jaundice and a feeling of "fullness" in the mid-epigastric area that radiates to his back. He states that this fullness never goes away, not even when he hasn't eaten for a long time. Current vitals are 102/62, 99.6, 88, and 28. His lab values are WBC 12,000, K 3.4, protein 4.8, albumin 2.9, AST 130, ALT 168, and LDH 225.

   a. You are the nurse assigned to this patient and you want a measurement of his abdominal girth. You know the significance of this measurement and ask the NAP to measure the patient's abdomen. Was this a good delegation?

   b. The patient now has to go for an MRI/CT scan. He needs to be NPO. The nurse asks the NAP to tell the patient that he is now NPO for the upcoming tests. Is this a good delegation?

   c. The patient's test results have come back, and lesions were found on his liver. The physician comes to the unit to biopsy the liver. It is now a few hours later, and a set of vitals needs to be taken for this patient. The nurse asks the NAP to get a set of vital signs. Is this a good delegation?

   d. The test results from the biopsy have come back, and the physician has just told the patient that there is nothing that can be done. The patient has a prognosis of less than six months to live. The doctor leaves, and the patient is all alone. The nurse asks the NAP to check to see if the patient is doing alright. Is this a good delegation?

EXPLORING THE WEB

1. Visit www.nursingpower.net for a collection of anecdotes and inspirational stories about the nursing profession.

2. Go to http://scholar.google.com. Type in "delegation in nursing." Select the most current articles to maintain your knowledge base of delegating.

3. Visit the Indiana Center for Evidence Based Nursing Practice Web site at www.ebnp.org. Click on "Evidence into Practice" and search for practice guidelines for delegation.

REFERENCES

American Association of Critical Care Nurses (AACN). (2004). *AACN Delegation Handbook*. Aliso Viejo, CA: Author.

American Nurses Association. (2005). *Code of ethics for nurses with interpretive statements*. Washington, DC: American Nurses Publishing.

American Nurses Association. (2007). *Registered nurses utilization of nursing assistive personnel in all settings*. Washington, DC: American Nurses Publishing.

American Nurses Association and National Council of State Boards of Nursing. (2006). *Joint statement on delegation*. Retrieved December 1, 2009, from www.ncsbn.org

Benner, P., Tanner, C. A., & Chesla, C. A. (1996). *Expertise in nursing practice: Caring clinical judgment and ethics*. New York, NY: Springer Publishing Company.

DuBrin, A. J. (2000). The Active Manager. South-Western Pub., United Kingdom: South-Western Pub.

Fisher, J. L., & Koch, J. V. (1996). *Presidential Leadership: Making a Difference*. Phoenix, AZ: Oryx Press.

Harvard ManageMentor® Delegating Tools. (2004). *Delegation skills checklist*. Boston, MA: Harvard Business School Publishing.

Hersey, P., Blanchard, K., & Natemeyer, W. (1979). Situational leadership, perception and impact of power. *Group and Organizational Studies, 4*, 418–428.

Miller, T., Maloney, R., & Maloney, P. (2008). Power. In P. Kelly (Ed.), *Nursing leadership & management* (2nd ed.) (pp. 170–173). Clifton Park, NY: Delmar Cengage Learning.

National Council of State Boards of Nursing. (1995). *Delegation: Concepts and decision-making process*. Chicago, IL: Author.

National Council of State Boards of Nursing. (1997). *Delegation decision-making tree.* Chicago, IL: Author.

National Council of State Boards of Nursing. (2007). *Medication Assistant-Certified (MA-C) model curriculum.* Retrieved September 7, 2007, from www.ncsbn.org

Nursing and Nurse Midwifery Council. (2008, May). *Advice for delegation for registered nurses and nurse midwives.* Retrieved from December 1, 2009, from www.nmc-uk.org

SUGGESTED READINGS

Currie, P. (2008). Delegation considerations for nursing practice. *Critical Care Nurse, 28*(5), 86–87.

Hancock, H., Campbell, S., Ramprogus, V., & Kilgour, J. (2008). Role development in health care assistants: The impact of education on practice. *Journal of Evaluation in Clinical Practice, 11*(5), 489–498.

Henderson, D., Sealover, P., Sharrer, V., Fusner, S., Sweet, S., & Blake, T. (2006). Nursing EDGE: Evaluating delegation guidelines in education. *International Journal of Nursing Education Scholarship, 3*(1), article 15.

McInnis, L. A., & Parsons, L. C. (2009). Thoughtful nursing practice: Reflections on nurse delegation decision-making. *Nursing Clinics of North America, 44*(4), 461–470.

National Council of State Boards of Nursing. (2004). *Model nursing practice act and rules.* Retrieved December 1, 2009, from www.ncsbn.org

O'Keefe, D. (2005, January/February). State laws and regulations for dialysis: An overview. *Nephrology Nursing Journal, 32*(1), 31–37.

Quallich, S. (2005). A bond of trust: Delegation. *Urologic Nursing, 25*(2), 120–123.

Reinhard, S., Young, H., Kane, R., & Quinn, W. (2006). Nurse delegation of medication administration for older adults in assisted living. *Nurse Outlook, 54*(2), 74–80.

Rowe, A. R., Savigny, D., Lanata, C., & Victora, C. G. (2005). How can we achieve and maintain high-quality performance of health workers in low-resources settings? *Lancet, 366,* 1026–1035.

CHAPTER 3
Effective Communication

Maureen T. Marthaler, Jacklyn L. Ruthman,
Crisamar Javellana-Anunciado, Paul Heidenthal,
Patricia Kelly

A nurse is the most profound fulcrum between the patient and the care they require. And it is the intimacy of the bedside nurse that effects the most powerful leverage of all.
—Ian Miller, RN

OBJECTIVES

Upon completion of this chapter, the reader should be able to:

1. Analyze how current trends in society affect communication.

2. Identify elements of the communication process.

3. Focus on the use of communication skills in delegation.

4. Discuss the impact of culture on delegation.

5. Review the professional role of the nurse.

6. Review potential barriers to communication.

7. Discuss various roles in communication.

8. Identify Myers-Briggs Personality Types.

9. Discuss workplace communication including communicating with superiors and other practitioners.

10. Discuss crew resource management.

As an RN working on an adult medical-surgical unit, you begin your shift by making patient rounds to perform initial assessments on your patients. Mr. Summer, who has a long history of hypertension, was admitted last night with complications. He is well known to the experienced staff. As you assess his breath sounds, he tells you with eyes downcast, "I don't think I'm going to make it this time." His wife, who is at his bedside, replies, "Don't talk like that."

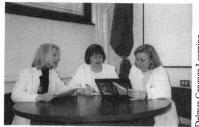

What are your thoughts about this situation?

What communication skills will you use to respond appropriately?

How can you and your staff demonstrate caring behavior to Mr. Summer and his wife?

Today's nurses use basic principles of communication to facilitate interactions with patients, family members, other nurses and health care providers, and professionals in other disciplines. These principles allow nurses to adapt to trends that affect the profession of nursing and its practice. Nurses use communication skills to effectively delegate patient care to others. This chapter will discuss elements of the communication process, the impact of culture on delegation, potential barriers to communication, the Myers-Briggs Personality Types, and workplace communication. It will review the professional role of the nurse and crew resource management.

TRENDS IN SOCIETY THAT AFFECT COMMUNICATION

Good communication will grow in importance because of trends in our culture. Among the trends affecting nursing practice is the increasing diversity in society. The United States has been called "the melting pot," and that has never been more true than now as we increasingly see the influence of many different ethnic, racial, cultural, and socioeconomic backgrounds. Increased diversity causes once-dominant values and beliefs to be replaced or diluted with different values and beliefs. These differences become a source of possible misunderstanding that can be bridged by effective communication.

Another trend is our aging population. It is estimated that 20% of the population will be 65 years of age or older by 2020. Our aging society will challenge nurses to maintain effective communication to compensate for the diminished sensory abilities that typically accompany aging. Multiple sensory deficits can occur simultaneously so that patients may experience losses in a variety of combinations that include hearing, seeing, smelling, tasting, and touching. This diminished input challenges nurse and patient alike to creatively compensate for these deficits. At the same time as the population is aging, it is also shifting to an electronic mode, with computer technology playing an increasingly dominant role. As electronic communication assumes a greater role, the nurse's ability to effectively communicate in writing will grow in importance. Reliance on written communication using electronic input shifts the source of input away from traditional visual, auditory, and kinesthetic modes to the written word. To use electronic tools effectively, tomorrow's nurses will require keen writing skills. These trends have influenced nursing today.

ELEMENTS OF THE COMMUNICATION PROCESS

Communication is an interactive process that occurs when a person (the sender) sends a verbal or nonverbal message to another person (the receiver) and receives feedback. The communication process is influenced by emotions, needs, perceptions, values, education, culture, goals, literacy, cognitive ability, and the communication mode. See Figure 3-1. The communication relayed from the sender to the receiver can include useful, distasteful, good, or bad information.

Written communication in nursing can be transmitted through a patient assignment sheet. The written assignment sheet provides the nurses and nursing assistive personnel (NAP) with a list of patients for whom they will care. The written assignment sheet transmits information as to who is to do what for a particular shift.

All aspects of communication are relevant to patient care. Accrediting agencies have developed standards to protect patients, as they have observed that a lack of communication can play an integral role in the occurrence of a sentinel event resulting in the death of, or serious physical or psychological injury to, a patient. While setting standards obviously cannot ensure good communication and coordination of patient care, the need to set standards does symbolize the growing recognition among accrediting and other oversight bodies that communication and coordination is highly important to the performance of health care organizations (Munoz & Luckmann, 2005).

Communication in health care is used to coordinate patient care. Several studies of ICUs indicate that effective communication and coordination among clinical staff results in more efficient and better quality of care (Baggs, Ryan, Phelps, Richeson, & Johnson, 1992; Knaus, Draper, Wagner, & Zimmerman, 1986; Shortell et al., 1994). More recent studies of other health care delivery settings also indicate that effective coordination of staff

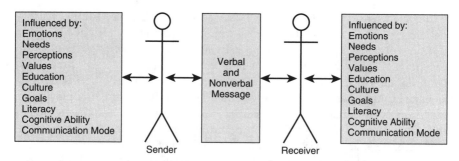

Figure 3-1 Communication process. (Delmar Cengage Learning.)

leads to better clinical outcomes (Gittell et al., 2000; Young et al., 1997). Additionally, research suggests that ineffective coordination and communication among hospital staff contributes substantially to adverse events (Andrews et al., 1997).

COMMUNICATION SKILLS AND DELEGATION

Communication is a cornerstone to achieving success when delegating patient care. Optimal patient outcomes are achieved when the initial directions of the nurse clearly define the expectations for the NAP or licensed practical nurse/licensed vocational nurse (LPN/LVN) in performing the assigned task. The use of the "four Cs" in giving initial directions can help improve the communication of delegated tasks (Zerwekh & Claborn, 2009). See Table 3-1.

A common pitfall when working with individuals for long periods of time is that people fall into routines. When this happens, the amount of talking may decrease and unrealistic expectations can occur. This can be positive or negative for the patient. The Joint Commission (JC) announces National Patient Safety Goals yearly. Included in the goals can be recommendations on improving communication among staff. The Joint Commission's goals can be found on their Web site at www.jointcommission.org.

The main reason for emphasizing effective communication is clear. Safe, quality patient care is compromised when lack of clear communication occurs among those providing care. Examples such as "I thought you said . . ." or "Didn't I ask you to let me know how the procedure went?" or "Well, that isn't what I meant . . . ," not to mention "Nobody ever told me to do it that way . . . ," are classic examples of comments people make when communication has broken down.

The nurse must ask three questions in seeking effective communication: (1) Was there a sender and a receiver for the communication?,

TABLE 3-1
FOUR CS OF COMMUNICATION

CLEAR	Does the team member understand what I am saying?
CONCISE	Have I confused the direction by giving too much unnecessary information?
CORRECT	Is the direction given according to policy, procedure, job description, and the law?
COMPLETE	Does the team member have all the information necessary to complete the task?

Adapted from *Nursing Today: Transition and Trends* (6th ed.), by J. Zerwekh and J. Claborn, 2009, St. Louis, Missouri: Saunders.

(2) Was the communication received?, and (3) Did the communication change behavior and result in the intended outcome? The answer to all three questions must be "yes" if communication is to be successful.

INTERPERSONAL COMMUNICATION

Interpersonal communication involves communication between individuals, whether person to person or in small groups. Not surprisingly, nurses engage in this type of communication regularly. The nurse who observes a patient grimace when he moves interprets this nonverbal cue as indicating that the patient is experiencing pain. Using verbal communication, she clarifies her perception by asking the patient to describe and rate his pain. He describes it as tolerable and states he is expecting a visitor and does not want to be drowsy. The communication goes back and forth until, ideally, both parties' understanding of the message match. This is the goal of communication. Note that good nursing care and effective nursing and medical practitioner communication has been linked to patient survival in ICUs (Arford, 2005).

COMMUNICATION SKILLS

Effective communication requires that both parties use communication skills that enhance a particular interaction. Baker, Beglinger, King, Salyards, and Thompson (2000) believe that the most important considerations to facilitate communication are to be open and willing to give and receive feedback. Some important skills nurses rely on to facilitate communication are attending, responding, clarifying, and confronting. See Table 3-2.

TABLE 3-2
COMMUNICATION SKILLS

Skill	Description
Attending	Active listening for what is said and how it is said, as well as noting of nonverbal cues that support or negate congruence; for example, making eye contact and posturing
Responding	Verbally and nonverbally acknowledging the sender's message, such as "I hear you"
Clarifying	Restating, questioning, and rephrasing to help the message become clear; for example, "I lost you there"
Confronting	Identifying the conflict; for example, "We have a problem here," and then clearly delineating the problem. Confronting uses knowledge and reason to resolve the problem
Supporting	Siding with another person or backing up another person: "I can see why you would feel that way"
Focusing	Centering on the main point: "So your main concern is..."
Open-ended questioning	Allowing for patient-directed responses: "How did that make you feel?"
Providing information	Supplying one with knowledge he or she did not previously have: "It's common for people with pneumonia to be tired"
Using silence	Allowing for intrapersonal communication
Reassuring	Restoring confidence or removing fear: "I can assure you that tomorrow..."
Expressing appreciation	Showing gratitude: "Thank you" or "You are so thoughtful"
Using humor	Providing relief and gaining perspective; may also cause harm, so use carefully
Conveying acceptance	Making known that one is capable or worthy: "It's okay to cry"
Asking related questions	Expanding listener's understanding: "How painful was it?"

Adapted from *Personal and Interdisciplinary Communication* by J. Ruthman. In *Nursing leadership & management* (2nd ed.) (pp. 123–131) by P. Kelly, 2008, Clifton Park, NY: Delmar Cengage Learning.

REAL WORLD INTERVIEW

I view my primary responsibility as a nurse to be that of patient advocate. As a team leader, I am responsible for coordinating patient care for a group of patients. I am responsible for setting patient care goals and then directing my team to achieve the goals. I make those patient care goals the focus of my team's efforts. Patient care is rendered with the assistance of subordinates, including nursing assistive personnel (NAP), nursing student externs, and occasional high school student volunteers. Communication is the key to a successful team. The following patient interaction typifies how I interact with my team.

An elderly nonverbal patient with a history of schizophrenia was admitted to our surgical unit for dehydration. She was in need of total care—especially with respect to hygiene, which had been neglected. She was dependent on staff to turn and position her. Her level of awareness suggested she was unable to use a call light for help.

This patient challenged staff for a variety of reasons. First, due to multiple other health problems, she was not a candidate for surgery. This placed her among the patients who don't really "fit" the surgical unit where she was admitted. Nonetheless, my goal was to advocate for comfort care with her physician while also encouraging subordinates to provide quality care, even though we could not cure this particular patient. The patient's inability to communicate verbally added to the challenge. It was unclear how aware the patient was of the care she was receiving. Her nonverbal status blocked her ability to dialogue. This caused us to rely on nonverbal cues. Respect for patients with or without their verbal feedback is essential. The NAP and I tackled the bed bath together. Teamwork kept the focus on the goal for the patient, which was to optimize comfort and maintain skin integrity. It allowed me to complete a thorough assessment and to model desired communication with the patient, whom I addressed by name. I inquired whether she was in pain, to which she responded with twisting motions. I continued the one-way conversation, attempting to clarify what her nonverbal responses meant. She pointed to her shoulder, so we repositioned her and she settled down, resting quietly. As is often the case, the NAP willingly returned to reposition the patient with confidence the remainder of the shift. The patient's inability to verbalize needs was perceived as less of a barrier once we were successful in overcoming it together.

I find that NAP will often volunteer to complete entire tasks when I have supported them and they feel capable of performing them independently. They must also have confidence that they will not be expected to handle clinical situations for which they do not feel qualified. They are required to honor the standard of care and will often complete tasks, going above and beyond what I ask. For example, later in the afternoon, the NAP returned to the patient and washed and braided her hair.

(continues)

Real World Interview *(continued)*

Since this patient would not likely use the call light, I also explained our goal to the high school student volunteer and I asked her to check the patient's position whenever she went by the room. I instructed her to let me know if the patient appeared uncomfortable, assuring her that I would reposition the patient as needed. The student expressed that she thought it was cool how nurses communicate with patients who can't talk. I believe through effective communication our team achieved the goal of optimizing this patient's comfort in spite of many potential barriers.

Lari Summa, RN, BSN

Attending.   **Attending** involves active listening. Active listening requires that the nurse pay close attention to what the patient is communicating, both verbally and nonverbally. The nurse pays close attention during communication, looking for congruence between what is said and how it is said. Attending involves the nurse's nonverbal cues. Facing the patient and maintaining eye contact are two skills that facilitate attending. If possible, sitting down and leaning forward sends a message that the nurse is willing to listen. Distracting behaviors, such as tapping one's foot, send a message that the nurse is not interested in the patient's message. Therefore, these types of behaviors should be avoided.

Responding.   **Responding** entails verbal and nonverbal acknowledgment of the sender's message. When the nurse nods affirmatively while listening, he or she communicates nonverbally that the sender's message has worth. A response can be as simple as an acknowledgment that the message was received, e.g., "I hear you." Sometimes, however, responding involves more. Two verbal skills that elevate the level of responding are questioning and restating. Questioning allows the nurse to clarify the message by asking related questions. Restating involves repeating what the nurse believes to be the important points. These techniques refine perceptions and enhance understanding.

Clarifying.   **Clarifying** helps the communication become clear through the use of such techniques as restating and questioning. For example, if the nurse does not understand a patient's account of a presenting complaint, the nurse can respond with, "I lost you there." Perhaps the nurse is trying to process information that is confusing or conflicting. He or she can restate what was heard in an effort to clarify the information. Questioning and restating are used not only to respond, but also to clarify.

Confronting. **Confronting** means to work jointly with others to resolve a problem or conflict. Given this definition, it is a very effective means of resolving conflict. See the discussion of conflict later in this chapter. Confronting involves, first of all, identifying the conflict, which can arise from perceived or real differences. A nurse might identify a conflict with a simple, "We have a problem here." Next, the problem is clearly delineated so that those involved understand what it is and what it is not. Then, using knowledge and reason, attempts are made to resolve the problem. The goal is to achieve a win-win solution where both parties' needs are met. This sounds easier to do than it sometimes is because emotions can get in the way and cloud reason. Cooling-off periods are sometimes needed between problem identification and conflict resolution. Acceptable motives for confronting are to resolve conflict, to further growth, and to improve relationships (Ruthman, 2008).

KEEP YOUR PATIENTS SAFE 3-1

The nursing assistive personnel (NAP), a student about to graduate from nursing school, is asked to help Mr. Jones move to the chair. As the NAP prepares to transfer Mr. Jones from the bed to the chair, the patient complains of a severe headache. He looks at the NAP and inquires, "I thought I was supposed to lie flat for one more hour?" The NAP immediately returns the patient to the supine position and goes to the nurse. The NAP tells the nurse that the patient has a severe headache and said that he thought he was supposed to lie flat for one more hour. The nurse says to the NAP, "I did not mean *that* Mr. Jones; I meant the Mr. Jones who is in room 345." The nurse immediately went to assess the patient with the headache. The NAP was unaware the patient with a headache recently underwent a lumbar puncture.

Why did this poor communication happen?

How could this incident have been prevented?

CULTURE AND DELEGATION

Culture encompasses different groups' beliefs and practices by gender, race, age, economic status, health, and disability (Ruthman, 2008). Our culture is becoming increasingly diverse. This diversity reduces the likelihood that patients, nurses, and other health care staff will share a common cultural background. In turn, the number of safe assumptions about beliefs and practices decreases and the probability for misunderstanding increases. Giger and Davidhizar (2008) outline six phenomena that must be considered when delegating to staff with culturally diverse backgrounds. These phenomena are communication, space, social organization, time, environmental control, and biological variations. See Table 3-3.

TABLE 3-3

CONSIDER THESE CULTURAL PHENOMENA AS YOU
DELEGATE PATIENT CARE TO STAFF

Phenomena	Example
Communication	Consider cultural communication elements such as communication volume, dialect, use of touch, context of speech, and kinesics such as gestures, stance, and eye behavior as you delegate patient care to staff.
Space	Consider physical closeness as you delegate patient care to staff. Some cultures prefer to stand physically close while communicating. Others prefer to maintain more physical distance between themselves and others.
Social Organization	When communicating, recognize that cultures vary in the amount of close social supports they maintain with family and others, including social support maintained with other health care staff.
Time	Cultures vary in their past, present, and future orientation. Note that some cultures focus on maintaining past traditions, other cultures focus on current activities, and still other cultures focus on preparing for the future.
Environmental Control	Note that cultures with an internal locus of control plan and take action. They don't rely on luck or fate. Cultures with an external locus of control wait for fate and luck to determine and guide their actions.
Biological Variations	Note that there are cultural biological variations in such things as physiological strength, stamina, and susceptibility to disease. Consider these as you delegate patient care to staff.

COMMUNICATION

Communication, the first cultural phenomenon, is greatly affected by cultural diversity in the work force. Elements of communication, such as dialect, volume, use of touch, context of speech, and kinesics (such as gestures, stance, and eye behavior), all influence how messages are sent and received (Giger & Davidhizar, 2008). For example, if a nurse is talking to a NAP in a loud voice, that might be interpreted as anger. However, the nurse may be from a cultural background in which people typically speak loudly. The nurse may not be angry at all. Alternatively, a nurse, because of cultural upbringing, may speak in a quiet, nondirective way that could be wrongly perceived as lacking authority.

SPACE

Cultural background influences the space that individuals maintain between themselves and others. Some cultures prefer physical closeness when speaking, whereas other cultures prefer more distance to be maintained between people. Ineffective delegation can take place when an individual's space is violated. Some people stand too close to others when speaking. Conversely, some people may feel left out if they are not sitting close to the delegator. They may not feel included or important.

SOCIAL ORGANIZATION

In different cultures, the social support in a person's life varies from support from one's own family, friends, and environment to support from collegial relationships within the workplace. If a staff member looks to other staff at work for social support, those staff may have difficulty fulfilling any tasks delegated to them that could threaten their social support or organization.

TIME

Another cultural phenomenon affecting delegation is the concept of time. Have you heard someone say in referring to others, "They are on their own time schedule?" Some people tend to react and move more slowly, whereas other people move quickly and are prompt in meeting deadlines.

Giger and Davidhizar (2008) describe different cultural groups as being past-, present-, or future-oriented. Past-oriented cultures focus largely on their tradition and its maintenance. For example, these cultures invest much time preparing food that is traditional even though the food can be bought prepared in a store. Present-oriented cultures focus on day-to-day activity. For example, a present-oriented culture works hard for today's wages but does not plan for the future. Future-oriented cultures worry about what might happen in the future and prepare diligently for a potential problem, perhaps financial or health-related. A nurse delegator should always communicate not only the duties to be completed but also their deadline, so all personnel can perform their tasks in a timely fashion.

ENVIRONMENTAL CONTROL

Giger and Davidhizar (2008) define environmental control as people's perception of control over their environment. Some cultures place a heavy emphasis on fate, luck, or chance, believing, for example, that a patient is cured from cancer based on chance. They may think the health care treatment had something to do with the cure, but was not the sole or even primary cause of the cure. They may stress the role of fate as an external locus of control.

How staff perceives their control of the environment may affect how they delegate and perform duties. Staff with an internal locus of control are geared toward setting goals, taking more control, having self-initiative, and not requiring assistance in decision making. They believe in taking action and not relying on fate.

Staff with an external locus of control may wait for others, or luck or fate, to determine their actions and tell them what to do. The nurse delegator working with this group must spell out very clearly what the staff must complete.

KEEP YOUR PATIENTS SAFE 3-2

The Luck Factor: The Four Essential Principles, published in 2004, authored by R. Wiseman, discusses research that illustrates luck as something that can be learned if one pays attention to four principles:
• Lucky people create, notice, and act on the opportunities in their life.
• Lucky people make successful decisions by using their intuition and gut feeling.
• Lucky people's expectations about the future help them fulfill their dreams and ambitions.
• Lucky people are able to transform their bad luck into good fortune.
Do you agree with Wiseman's findings? Can you use your "luck" to control your environment, set your goals, and improve your nursing career? Your life? Discuss.

BIOLOGICAL VARIATIONS

The sixth cultural phenomenon is biological variations. Biological variations are the biological differences between racial and ethnic groups. These biological variations include physiological differences, physical stamina, and susceptibility to disease. For example, the nursing care of a comatose patient who weighs more than 300 pounds and who requires frequent turning should not be delegated to a small nurse who can't physically handle the patient. Perhaps this patient should be assigned to two nurses. Likewise, a pregnant nurse should not be assigned to a patient with radium implants because of the risks radium may pose to the baby and mother. Biological variations must be considered for the sake of both the health care providers and their patients.

THE PROFESSIONAL ROLE OF THE NURSE

Nurses have a legal and professional responsibility to deliver quality nursing care to their patients. Experts in the social sciences are considered the authorities on what makes an occupation a profession. Although there is some variation in actual criteria of a profession, general agreement exists in several areas:

- Professional status is achieved when an occupation involves a unique practice that carries individual responsibility and is based upon theoretical knowledge.
- The privilege to practice is granted only after the individual has completed a standardized program of highly specialized education and has demonstrated an ability to meet the standards for practice.
- The body of specialized knowledge is continually developed and evaluated through research.
- The members are self-organizing, and they collectively assume the responsibility of establishing standards for education in practice. They continually evaluate the quality of services provided in order to protect the individual members and the public.

There is a trend in recent years to call every occupation a profession. Have you heard of professional computer operators, professional automobile mechanics, professional teachers, professional nurses, and professional lawyers? There has been a tendency to confuse "professionalism" and "profession." The term "professionalism" generally refers to an individual's commitment and dedication to his or her occupation. Professionalism often also refers to the attitude, appearance, and conduct of the individual. Whether an occupation is a profession requires more analysis. Figure 3-2 refers to some characteristics of a profession identified by different sources. Figure 3-3 lists some of the values, behaviors, and attributes that may be exhibited by a "professional." Table 3-4 identifies some tips for you to use as you develop your professional style.

Flexner, 1915	Bixler and Bixler, 1959
• Intellectual activities • Activities based on knowledge • Activities can be learned • Activities must be practical • Techniques are teachable • A strong organization exists • Altruism motivates the work	• Specialized body of knowledge • Growing body of knowledge • New knowledge used to improve education and practice • Education takes place in higher education institutions • Autonomous practice • Service above personal gain • Compensation through freedom of action, continuing professional growth, and economic security
Pavalko, 1971	**Public Law 93-360 on Collective Bargaining**
• Work based on systematic body of theory and abstract knowledge • Work has social value • Length of education required for specialization • Service to public • Autonomy • Commitment to profession • Group identity and subculture • Existence of a code of ethics	• Predominantly intellectual work • Varied work requirements • Requires discretion and judgment • Results cannot be standardized over time • Requires advanced instruction and study

Figure 3-2 Characteristics of a profession. (Courtesy *Nursing Perspectives and Issues* (5th ed.), by P. R. Mitchell and G. M. Grippando, 1994, Albany, NY: Delmar Publishers.)

FOUR ESSENTIAL DIMENSIONS OF NURSING

1. *Nursing* is the protection, promotion, and optimization of health and abilities, prevention of illness and injury, alleviation of suffering through the diagnosis and treatment of human response, and advocacy in the care of individuals, families, communities, and populations (American Nurses Association, 2003).
2. *Distinctive services* that nurses provide focus on the response of the individual and the family to actual or potential health problems. Nurses are educated to be attuned to the whole person, not just the unique

(continues)

Four Essential Dimensions of Nursing *(continued)*

presenting health problem. While a medical diagnosis of an illness may be fairly circumscribed, the human response to a health problem may be much more fluid and variable and may have a great effect on the individual's ability to overcome the initial medical problem. It is often said that physicians cure and nurses care. In what some describe as a blend of physiology and psychology, nurses build on their understanding of the disease and illness process to promote the restoration and maintenance of health in their clients (American Nurses Association, 2008).

3. *Benefits to consumers* include lower rates of nurse-sensitive outcomes (defined in research study as death of a patient with one of the following life-threatening complications: pneumonia, shock, cardiac arrest, urinary tract infection, gastrointestinal bleeding, sepsis, or deep vein thrombosis, and "failure to rescue") (Needleman, Buerhaus, Mattke, Stewart, & Zelevinsky, 2002).

4. *Costs of nursing services* vary according to the care setting and role of the nurse. Primary care delivered by nurse practitioners and services provided by certified nurse midwives cost less than the same care delivered by physicians (Shi & Singh, 2001).

Professional Values		
• Caring	• Freedom	• Justice
• Altruism	• Esthetics	• Truth
• Equality	• Human dignity	• Ethics
• Nonjudgmentalism		

Professional Behaviors and Attributes	
• Appearance	• Political awareness
• Time management skills	• Reading of professional journals
• Self-discipline	• Participation in nursing research
• Maintenance of licensure/ certification	• Stress management
• Participation in institutional/ community activities	• Self-evaluation
	• Initiative
• Participation in continuing education	• Motivation
	• Creativity
	• Effective communication

Figure 3-3 Possible characteristics of a professional. (Courtesy *Nursing Perspectives and Issues* (5th ed.), by P. R. Mitchell and G. M. Grippando, 1994, Albany, NY: Delmar Publishers.)

TABLE 3-4
DEVELOPING A PROFESSIONAL STYLE

1. What is your current education and experience?
2. Set goals for any additional education and experience that you may need.
3. As you start your new nursing role, review the following on your unit:
   • Ten most common medical diagnoses
   • Ten most common nursing diagnoses
   • Ten most common medications and IV solutions
   • Ten most common diagnostic tests
   • Ten most common laboratory tests
   • Ten most common nursing and medical interventions and treatments
4. Review your own job description and the role and the job description of nursing and other staff you work with.
5. Identify the names and contact information of all nursing, medical, and health care staff that you work with.
6. Discuss delegation with your preceptor and observe how the preceptor delegates to others.
7. Observe the impact of delegation on both the delegate and the person delegated to.
8. Remember the golden rule: Do unto others as you would want them to do unto you.
9. Recognize that, under the nurse practice act, the RN holds the responsibility and accountability for nursing care.
10. Practice assertiveness and work at being direct, open, and honest in your nursing role.
11. Exercise your power with kindness to all.
12. Hold others accountable and responsible for their duties as spelled out in their job description.
13. Be open to performance improvement feedback about your personal delegation style.
14. Modify your communication approach to fit the needs of patients, staff, and yourself.

POTENTIAL BARRIERS TO COMMUNICATION

The nurse who can identify potential barriers to communication will be better equipped to avoid them or to compensate for them. Some of the most common barriers in addition to culture are gender, anger, status differences, incongruent responses, conflict, and thought distortions. Other barriers to communication are listed in Table 3-5.

TABLE 3-5
ADDITIONAL BARRIERS TO COMMUNICATION

Barrier	Description
Offering false reassurance	Promising something that cannot be delivered
Being defensive	Acting as though one has been attacked
Stereotyping	Unfairly categorizing someone based on his or her traits
Interrupting	Speaking before the other person has completed his or her message
Inattention	Not paying attention
Stress	A state of tension that gets in the way of reasoning
Unclear expectations	Ill-defined direction to perform tasks or duties that makes successful completion of them unlikely
Incongruent responses	When words and actions in communication don't match the inner experience of self and/or are inappropriate to the context. This response commonly presents itself as blaming, placating, being super reasonable, or using irrelevant information when communicating with another person
Giving advice	Assumes the other person is unable to solve his or her own problems

Adapted from *Personal and Interdisciplinary Communication* by J. Ruthman. In *Nursing leadership & management* (2nd ed.) (pp. 123–131) by P. Kelly, 2008, Clifton Park, NY: Delmar Cengage Learning.

GENDER

Gender interferes with communication when men and women lack the understanding that they may process information differently. In general, some men are more interested in using communication to solve problems and get a task done. Some women talk to make a point, give and receive emotional support, relieve tension, or discover a point. Every person has a natural blend of masculine and feminine characteristics (Gray, 2001). Gender differences and patterns do not preclude men and women from working together. Rather, they require that both groups realize that the other may have different preferences and make accommodations so that effective communication and working relationships result.

Gender differences have been attributed, in part, to gender socialization, in which males may have been provided with more opportunities to develop confidence and assertiveness than females. The feminist movement and increased sexual equality in western society, in general, have weakened traditional sociological patterns of competitiveness and decisiveness in men and passivity and nurturing in women. However, remnants of the traditional model persist, particularly in health care settings. Nurses who lack assertiveness and confidence are encouraged to acquire the requisite skills to be assertive and confident in order to be an effective patient advocate and also to communicate in a confident manner (Ruthman, 2008).

ANGER

Anger is a universal, strong feeling of displeasure that is often precipitated by a situation that frustrates or prevents a person from attaining a goal. Anger is influenced by one's beliefs. Ellis (2002) describes anger as an irrational response that arises from one of four irrational ideas: (1) thinking that the treatment one received was awful (awfulizing), (2) feeling that one can't stand having been treated so irresponsibly and unfairly (can't-stand-it-itis), (3) believing that one should not, and must not behave as he or she did (shoulding and musting), and (4) thinking that because one acted in a terrible manner, he or she is a terrible person (undeservingness and damnation). See Table 3-6. Ellis maintains that beliefs remain rational as long as the evaluation of the action does not involve an evaluation of the person. Rational and appropriate responses include feelings of disappointment. Anger, on the other hand, can be unmanageable and self-defeating. Ellis believes that we all have the ability to choose our response to anger.

Anger can be dealt with in one of several ways. Three methods that may work from time to time but have serious and potentially destructive drawbacks are denying and repressing anger, which may lead to resentment; expressing anger, which may lead to defensiveness on the part of

TABLE 3-6
FOUR IRRATIONAL IDEAS WHICH LEAD TO ANGER
Awfulizing
Can't-stand-it-itis
Shoulding and musting
Undeservingness and damnation

Adapted from *Anger: How to live with and without it,* by A. Ellis, 2002, New York, NY: Kensington Publishing Corporation.

the respondent; and turning the other cheek, which may lead to continued mistreatment and lack of trust. Since anger stems from carrying things further and viewing the situation as awful, terrible, or horrible, Ellis (2002) advocates disputing irrational beliefs. Anger can stem from deep-seated feelings of unassertiveness. Assertion involves taking a stand, whereas aggression involves putting another person down. If unassertiveness is the source of anger, then a solution is to learn to act assertively.

STATUS DIFFERENCES

Status is the measure of worth conferred on an individual by a group. Status differences are seen throughout organizations and serve some useful purposes (Shortell & Kaluzny, 2006). Differences in status motivate people, provide them with a means of identification, and may be a force for stability in the organization (Scott, 1967).

Status differences have a profound effect on the functioning of teams. Research findings are fairly consistent in showing that high-status members initiate communication more often, are provided more opportunities to participate, and have more influence over the decision-making process (Owens, Mannic, & Neale, 1998). Thus, an individual from a lower-status professional group may be intimidated or ignored by higher-status team members. The group, as a result, may not benefit from this person's expertise. This situation is very likely in health care, where status differences among the professions are well entrenched (Topping, Norton, & Scafidi, 2003). Often, multidisciplinary teams are idealistically expected to operate as a company of equals, yet the reality of the situation makes this difficult (Shortell & Kaluzny, 2006). In a study of end-stage renal disease teams, in which the equal participation ideology was accepted by most team participants, it was clear that the medical practitioners, who were perceived as having higher professional status than other groups, had greater involvement in the actual decision-making process (Deber & Leatt, 1986). The mismatch between expectations and reality made many team members, particularly staff nurses, feel a sense of role deprivation, with accompanying implications for morale and job satisfaction. This problem is exacerbated in teams characterized by sex diversity. In one study, men were more likely to want to exit teams that were female-dominated for those that were male-dominated or homogeneous. Following from this, men have historically been perceived as having higher status in managerial roles in organizations, thereby affecting the men's satisfaction with the team (Chatman & O'Reilly, 2004).

Status differences may have very significant impacts on patient outcomes. According to the recent report, *Keeping Patients Safe: Transforming the Work Environment of Nurses,* "counterproductive hierarchical communication patterns that derive from status differences" are partly responsible for many medical errors (Institute of Medicine, 2003). Further, a review of medical malpractice cases from across the country found that medical practitioners, perceived by some as the higher-status members of the team, often ignored important information communicated by nurses, perceived by some as the lower-status members of the team. Nurses in turn were found to withhold relevant information for diagnosis and treatment from medical practitioners (Schmitt, 2001). In this status-conscious environment, opportunities for learning and improvement can be missed because of unwillingness to engage in quality-improving communication.

INCONGRUENT RESPONSES

When words and actions in communication don't match the inner experience of self and/or are inappropriate to the context, the response is incongruent. Some common incongruent responses are blaming, placating, being super reasonable, and using irrelevant information for decision making.

Blaming is finding fault or error and occurs when a response lacks respect for others' feelings. For example, a nurse who attributes a medication error to an overloaded assignment might blame the nurse who made the assignment, claiming that "It's all her fault." This can be avoided by speaking up when the assignment is made and standing up for one's rights while respecting the rights of others.

Placating is soothing by concession and occurs when one lacks self-respect. For example, a nurse who consents to a patient assignment that he or she believes is unfair or unsafe just to keep the peace is placating. Placating can be overcome by paying attention to one's own needs and by negotiating what one believes to be a fair and safe assignment.

Being super reasonable is to go beyond reason and demonstrate lack of respect for others' and one's own feelings. The nurse above, who when approached by the house supervisor agrees to whatever solution is offered, has become super reasonable when he or she says, "You're always right; I'll do whatever you need." This ineffective approach can be sidestepped by clarifying goals and yet considering each other's feelings when arriving at a solution.

Finally, using irrelevant information for decision making shows lack of respect for others' and one's own feelings. A nurse who challenges a colleague's abilities based solely on his or her out-of-work activities or political preference is using irrelevant information. Likewise, arguing against a colleague's ability to function as a charge nurse because of an incident that occurred a year prior during the nurse's orientation may be irrelevant. Respecting feelings and the context within which an event occurred can avert irrelevance (Ruthman, 2008).

CONFLICT

Conflict arises when ideas or beliefs are opposed. Not surprisingly, it occurs at different levels, such as the interpersonal and organizational level. Conflict resolution is another way to resolve conflict besides the confronting method discussed earlier in this chapter. In conflict resolution, the nature of the differences and the reasons for the differences are considered. Differences arise for an array of reasons. Variations in facts, goals, and methods to achieve the goals, values, or standards, as well as priorities, all contribute to these differences (Kinney & Hurst, 1979). Conflict resolution typically occurs using different approaches. See Table 3-7.

TABLE 3-7
SUMMARY OF CONFLICT RESOLUTION TECHNIQUES

Conflict Resolution Technique	Advantages	Disadvantages
Accommodating— smoothing or cooperating. One side gives in to the other side	One side is more concerned with an issue than the other side; stakes are not high enough for one group and that side is willing to give in	One side holds more power and can force the other side to give in; the importance of the stakes are not as apparent to one side as the other; can lead to parties feeling "used" if they are always pressured to give in
Avoiding—one side ignores the conflict	Does not make a big deal out of nothing; conflict may be minor in comparison to other priorities; allows tempers to cool	Conflict can become bigger than anticipated; source of conflict might be more important to one person or group than others
Collaborating—both sides work together to develop optimal outcomes	Best solution for the conflict and encompasses all important goals on each side	Takes a lot of time; requires commitment to success
Competing—forcing; the two or three sides are forced to compete for the goal	Produces a winner; good when time is short and stakes are high	Produces a loser; may leave anger and resentment on losing side

(continues)

Table 3-7 *(continued)*

Conflict Resolution Technique	Advantages	Disadvantages
Compromising— each side gives up something and gains something	No one should win or lose, but both should gain something; good for disagreements between individuals	May cause a return to the conflict if what is given up becomes more important than the original goal
Confronting— immediate and obvious movement to stop conflict at the very start	Does not allow conflict to take root; very powerful	May leave impression that conflict is not tolerated; may make a big deal out of nothing
Negotiating—high-level discussion that seeks agreement but not necessarily consensus	Stakes are very high and solution is rather permanent; often involves powerful groups	Agreements are permanent, even though each side has gains and losses

THOUGHT DISTORTIONS

Research on thinking processes has shown that people sometimes make mistakes in the way they perceive information and think about the world around them. For example, when people are somewhat depressed, their automatic thoughts are loaded with distorted thinking. If one can recognize these thought distortions, one can begin to turn life in a more positive direction. See Table 3-8.

TABLE 3-8 *THOUGHT DISTORTIONS*	
Thought Distortion	**Example**
All-or-nothing thinking: seeing things only in absolutes	If I leave this job, no one will respect me.
Overgeneralization: interpreting every small setback as a never-ending pattern of defeat	Everyone here is so smart; I'm a real loser.
Dwelling on negatives: ignoring multiple positive experiences	I made a mistake. I'm not good enough to be a nurse.

(continues)

Table 3-8 *(continued)*

Jumping to conclusions: assuming that others are reacting negatively without definite evidence	I don't know why I study. Everyone thinks I'm going to fail NCLEX anyway.
Pessimism: automatically predicting that things will turn out badly	It's only a matter of time before everything falls apart for me.
Reasoning from feeling: thinking that if one feels bad, one must be bad	My head hurts because I'm a bad person. I deserve it!
Obligations: living life around a succession of too many "shoulds," "shouldn'ts," "musts," "oughts," and "have tos"	I should marry Mike. Everyone likes him.

Compiled with information from *Psychiatric Mental Health Nursing* (4th ed.), by N. C. Frisch and L. E. Frisch, 2011, Clifton Park, NY: Delmar Cengage Learning.

OVERCOMING COMMUNICATION BARRIERS

DuBrin (2000) has identified nine strategies and tactics for overcoming communication barriers. See Table 3-9. In addition to these strategies, it is helpful to avoid groupthink.

AVOIDING GROUPTHINK

Effective leaders work to avoid groupthink. The concept of groupthink emerged from Janis' studies of high-level policy decisions by government leaders, including decisions about Vietnam, the Bay of Pigs, and the Korean War.

TABLE 3-9
OVERCOMING COMMUNICATION BARRIERS

Understand the receiver.	• Ask yourself, what's in it for the other person? • Work to develop understanding of the other person's needs.
Communicate assertively.	• Be direct. • Explain ideas clearly and with feeling. • Repeat important messages. • Use various communication channels, e.g., written, e-mail, verbal, and so on.
Use two-way communication.	• Ask questions. • Communicate face to face.

(continues)

Table 3-9 *(continued)*

Unite with a common vocabulary.	• Define the meaning of important terms, such as "high quality," so that everyone understands their meaning.
Elicit verbal and nonverbal feedback.	• Request and offer verbal feedback often. • Document important agreements. • Observe nonverbal feedback.
Enhance listening skills.	• Pay attention to what is said, to what is not said, and to nonverbal signals. • Continue listening carefully even when you don't like the message. • Give summary reflections to assure understanding; for example, "You say you are late giving medication because the pharmacy did not deliver meds on time." • Engage in concluding discussions, such as, "Has your unit been late with medications due to problems with pharmacy deliveries before?" • Ask questions to explore problems. • Paraphrase a speaker's words to decrease miscommunication, rather than blurting out questions as soon as the other person finishes speaking.
Be sensitive to cultural differences.	• Know that cultural communication barriers exist. • Show respect for all workers. • Minimize use of jargon specific to your culture. • Be sensitive to cultural etiquette, such as use of first names, eye contact, hand gestures, and personal appearance.
Be sensitive to gender differences.	• Be aware that men and women may have some differences in communication style; for instance, men may call attention to their accomplishments and women may tend to be more conciliatory when facing differences. • Know that male-female stereotypes often don't fit the person you are working with. • Avoid barriers by knowing that differences exist and don't take things personally. • Males can improve communication by showing more empathy and females by becoming more direct.
Engage in meta-communication.	• Communicate about your communication to resolve a problem, such as, "I'm trying to get through to you, but either you don't react to me or you get angry. What can I do to improve our communication?"

Adapted from *The Active Manager,* by A. J. DuBrin, 2000, United Kingdom: South Western Pub.

Groupthink occurs when the desire for harmony and consensus overrides members' rational efforts to appraise the situation. In other words, groupthink occurs when maintaining the pleasant atmosphere of the team implicitly becomes more important to members than reaching a good decision (Shortell & Kaluzny, 2006). There is a reduced willingness to disagree and challenge other's views in groupthink. Some of all of the following symptoms may indicate the presence of groupthink (Janis, 1972):

- *The illusion of invulnerability:* Team members may reassure themselves about obvious dangers and become overly optimistic and willing to take extraordinary risks.
- *Collective rationalization:* Teams may overlook blind spots in their plans. When confronted with conflicting information, the team may spend considerable time and energy refuting the information and rationalizing a decision.
- *Belief in the inherent morality of the team:* Highly cohesive teams may develop a sense of self-righteousness about their role that makes them insensitive to the consequences of decisions.
- *Stereotyping others:* Victims of groupthink hold biased, highly negative views of competing teams. They assume that they are unable to negotiate with other teams, and rule out compromise.
- *Pressures to conform:* Group members face severe pressure to conform to team norms and to team decisions. Dissent is considered abnormal and may lead to formal or informal punishment.
- *The use of mindguards:* Mindguards are used by members who withhold or discount dissonant information that interferes with the team's current view of a problem.
- *Self-censorship:* Teams subject to groupthink pressure members to remain silent about possible misgivings and to minimize self-doubts about a decision.
- *Illusion of unanimity:* A sense of unanimity emerges when members assume that silence and lack of protest signify agreement and consensus.

Shortell and Kaluzny (2006) state that the consequences of groupthink are that teams may limit themselves, often prematurely, to one possible solution and fail to conduct a comprehensive analysis of a problem. When groupthink is well entrenched, members may fail to review their decisions in light of new information or changing events. Teams may also fail to consult adequately with experts within or outside the organization, and fail to develop contingency plans in the event that the decision turns out to be wrong.

Team leaders can help avoid groupthink. First, leaders can encourage members to critically evaluate proposals and solutions. When a leader is particularly powerful and influential, yet still wants to get unbiased views from team members, the leader may refrain from stating his or her own position until later in the decision-making process. Another strategy is to assign the same problem to two separate work teams. Most importantly, groupthink can be avoided by proactively engaging in a process of critical appraisal of ideas and solutions, and by understanding the warning signs of groupthink (Shortell & Kaluzny, 2006).

ROLES IN COMMUNICATION

In any group, there are bound to be both participants who are helpful and those who are not helpful in their behaviors. Sometimes these behaviors are unconsciously acted out. At other times, a group member is quite clear and focused about the role that he or she is playing, such as the aggressor. In any case, it is imperative that the astute nurse leader be aware of everyone's roles and use excellent communication skills to facilitate the team's work. See Table 3-10.

TABLE 3-10
COMMON MEMBER ROLES

Common member roles in groups fit into three categories: group task roles, group maintenance roles, and self-oriented roles.
- *Group task roles* help a group develop and accomplish its goals. Among these roles are the following:
  - Initiator-contributor: Proposes goals, suggests ways of approaching tasks, and recommends procedures for approaching a problem or task
  - Information seeker: Asks for information, viewpoints, and suggestions about the problem or task
  - Information giver: Offers information, viewpoints, and suggestions about the problem or task
  - Coordinator: Clarifies and synthesizes various ideas in an effort to tie together the work of the members
  - Orienter: Summarizes, points to departures from goals, and raises questions about discussion direction
  - Energizer: Stimulates the group to higher levels of work and better quality
- *Group maintenance roles* do not directly address a task itself but, instead, help foster group unity, positive interpersonal relations among group members, and development of the ability of members to work effectively together. Group maintenance roles include the following:
  - Encourager: Expresses warmth and friendliness toward group members, encourages them, and acknowledges their contributions
  - Harmonizer: Mediates disagreements between other members and attempts to help reconcile differences

(continues)

Table 3-10 *(continued)*

- ○ Gatekeeper: Tries to keep lines of communication open and promotes the participation of all members
- ○ Standard setter: Suggests standards for ways in which the group will operate and checks whether members are satisfied with the functioning of the group
- ○ Group observer: Watches the internal operations of the group and provides feedback about how participants are doing and how they might be able to function better
- ○ Follower: Goes along with the group and is friendly but relatively passive
- *Self-oriented roles* are related to the personal needs of group members and often negatively influence the effectiveness of a group. These roles include the following:
  - ○ Aggressor: Deflates the contributions of others by attacking their ideas, ridiculing their feelings, and displaying excessive competitiveness
  - ○ Blocker: Tends to be negative, stubborn, and resistive of new ideas, sometimes in order to force the group to readdress a viewpoint that it has already dealt with
  - ○ Recognition seeker: Seeks attention, boasts about accomplishments and capabilities, and works to prevent being placed in an inferior position in the group
  - ○ Dominator: Tries to assert control and manipulates the group or certain group members through such methods as flattering, giving orders, or interrupting others

Adapted from *Management* (3rd ed.), by K. Bartol and D. Martin, 1998, Boston, MA: McGraw-Hill.

DESTRUCTIVE OR DIFFICULT BEHAVIORS

Nurses who delegate may occasionally work with people who are not interested in good communication and accomplishing a task. Strategies for coping with these difficult people are identified in Table 3-11.

Other destructive behaviors that people on a health care team may exhibit include being the disapprover or blocker of others' suggestions; being a recognition seeker; being a self-confessor of personal, nongroup-oriented feelings or comments; being a playboy or playgirl; being a dominator or help seeker; or using the group to meet personal needs or to plead special interests (Northouse & Northouse, 1997). These destructive behaviors can interfere with the health care team's ability to meet the patient's needs.

TABLE 3-11
STRATEGIES FOR COPING WITH DIFFICULT PEOPLE

Personality Type	Coping Strategies
Criticizer	Don't argue—it will only add fuel to the fire! Ask for input and practice active listening by reflecting on what you heard. Give criticizers a project to which they can directly contribute.
Passive person	Engage in communication, ask direct questions, and ask for direct responses.
Detailer	Allow the detailer to give details at certain points in a group. Begin with the objective for the group, repeat information when necessary, summarize.
Controller	Keep focused on the task at hand; note any inconsistencies in the controller's conversation.
Pleaser	Let pleasers know that their comments are safe from attack, and that their opinions are valued.

Adapted from Polifko-Harris. In *Nursing leadership & management* (2nd ed.), by P. L. Kelly, 2008, Clifton Park, NY: Delmar Cengage Learning.

EVIDENCE FROM THE LITERATURE

Citation: Longo, J., & Sherman, R. O. (2007, March). Leveling horizontal violence. *Nursing Management, 38*(3), 34–37.

Discussion: Horizontal violence has been described as an expression of oppressed group behavior rooted in feelings of low self-esteem and lack of respect from others. Despite recent research that indicates a significant improvement in RNs' perceptions of satisfaction with their careers and work environments, the majority of nurses deny that nursing is a good career for people who want respect in their jobs. Nurses have been described as an oppressed group because the profession is primarily female and has existed under a historically patriarchal system headed by male physicians, administrators, and marginalized nurse managers.

Horizontal violence between nurses is an act of aggression perpetrated by one colleague toward another colleague. Although horizontal violence usually consists of verbal or emotional abuse, it can also include physical abuse and may be subtle or overt. Acts of horizontal violence can include talking behind one's back, belittling or criticizing a colleague

(continues)

Evidence from the Literature *(continued)*

in front of others, blocking information or a chance for promotion, and isolating or freezing a colleague out of group activities. Repeated acts of horizontal violence against another are often referred to as "bullying."

Common behaviors characterized as horizontal violence include

- Nonverbal behaviors, such as the raising of eyebrows or making faces, in response to comments from the victim
- Verbal remarks that could be characterized as being snide, or abrupt responses to questions raised by the victim
- Activities that undermine the victim's ability to perform professionally, including either refusing or not being available to give assistance
- The withholding of information about a practice or patient that will undermine a victim's ability to perform professionally
- Acts of sabotage that deliberately set victims up for negative situations in their work environment
- Group infighting and establishing of cliques designed to exclude some staff members
- Scapegoating or attributing all that goes wrong in a situation to one individual
- Failure to resolve conflicts directly with the individual involved, choosing instead to complain to others about an individual's behavior
- Failure to respect the privacy of others
- Broken confidences

Implications for Practice: Nurses can work to recognize horizontal violence in the profession. As horizontally violent behaviors are recognized, they can be eliminated.

MYERS-BRIGGS PERSONALITY TYPES

If a team is to succeed, it is helpful to have the right blend of personalities, experience, and temperaments to work toward a common goal. An astute nursing team leader will keep in mind that some personality types complement others. A tool that some organizations use to assist them in devising effective teams and team building is the Myers-Briggs Type Indicator® (MBTI), a psychological testing instrument that identifies different personality types (Figure 3-4). Major personality types according to the MBTI fall into four pairs of categories and indicate how people

1. Focus their attention: Are they an Introvert (I) or an Extrovert (E)?
2. Take in information from their surroundings: Are they Sensing (S) or Intuitive (N)?
3. Prefer to make decisions: Are they Thinking (T) or Feeling (F)?
4. Relate to the external world: Do they have Judging (J) characteristics or Perceiving (P) characteristics?

The MBTI categorizes individuals into each one of these four pairs of categories, for example, a person may be an Extrovert, Sensing, Feeling, Judging Type (ESFJ), or any one of sixteen different possible combinations of the four category pairs.

A critical point to make in using the MBTI is that in the MBTI, there is no right or wrong personality type. Everyone is different and these differences should be respected (Keirsey & Bates, 1978). The MBTI should only be used for guidance, not for placing people into distinct categories. In fact, most people are not at one end of the continuum or the other. Most are somewhere on a scale. For example, a person may be 60% Extrovert and 40% Introvert, 20% Sensing and 80% Intuitive, 90% Thinking and 10% Feeling, and 30% Judging and 70% Perceiving. The MBTI just provides one additional piece of information about people. Its results are not "locked in stone."

WORKPLACE COMMUNICATION

How individuals communicate depends, in part, on where communication occurs and in what relationship. Patterns of communication in the workplace are sensitive to organizational factors that define relationships. Nurses have diverse roles and relationships in the workplace that call for different communication patterns with superiors, co-workers, and other nursing and medical practitioners.

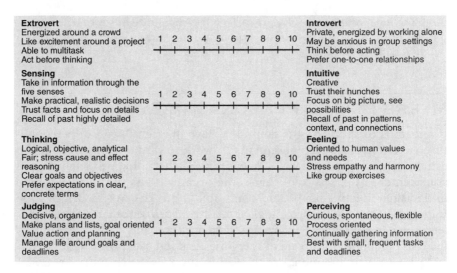

Figure 3-4 Myers-Briggs personality dichotomies. (Compiled from *Gifts Differing,* by B. M. Isabel and P. B. Myers, 1995, Palo Alto, CA: Davies-Black, and *Patient Teaching* by P. Kelly. In *Essentials of Nursing Leadership & Management* (2nd ed.), by P. Kelly, 2010, Clifton Park, NY: Delmar Cengage Learning.)

CASE STUDY 3-1

Nurses use routine standards to deliver quality patient care, maintain patient safety, and prevent nursing-sensitive patient outcomes. Examples of routine standards on all patient care units might include passing fresh water, giving morning care and baths, passing medications, monitoring vital signs, maintaining IV fluids and maintaining oral intake, etc. On a surgical unit, the routine standards might include such things as turning, coughing, and deep breathing patients every two hours, checking their bowel sounds, checking voiding, getting their legs moving, etc. Throughout the day shift, nursing and unit staff communicate and work together to deliver quality patient care according to a schedule something like this:

7:00 a.m.   Handoff shift report from night shift to day shift

7:15 a.m.   Charge nurse reviews patient care assignments with all nurses and unit staff; goals and priorities are set

7:20 a.m.   Ongoing patient assessment begins, i.e., assess patients ABCs, safety, comfort, infection control, vital signs, and diagnostic tests needed; maintain IV fluids; pass fresh water; keep siderails up; etc.

7:30 a.m.   Breakfast

7:45 a.m.   Morning care with bathing begins following nursing care standards and unit routines

8:00 a.m.   Medications given; medical and nursing practitioners make rounds; review all new orders; complete diagnostic tests and documentation; turn, cough, and deep breathe patients every two hours and check their breath sounds, bowel sounds, and voiding; keep patients' legs moving; ambulate patients; etc.

11:30 a.m.   Vital sign assessment

12:00 p.m.   Lunch; continue administering medications and other routine care

2:00 p.m.   Intake and output reports, and documentation completed

3:00 p.m.   Handoff shift report from day shift to evening shift

How does teamwork get patient care completed on a clinical unit? Does patient care on your clinical unit follow a similar time sequence as the routine standard above? Develop a routine standard for a group of patients at the front of this book. What elements did you include?

COMMUNICATING WITH SUPERVISORS

Communicating with supervisors about problems can be intimidating, especially for a new nurse. Observing professional courtesies is an important first step. For instance, if there is time, begin by requesting an appointment to discuss a problem. This demonstrates respect for the supervisor and allows for the conversation to occur at an appropriate time and place. If a problem is more pressing, report it to your supervisor as soon as possible. This report usually starts with the charge nurse, who may in turn need to communicate the problem to his or her supervisor. Don't hesitate to communicate up the organizational chain of command discussed in Chapter 1 if you feel the problem remains unresolved. It is usually best to start with your direct supervisor. Be prepared to state the concern clearly and accurately. Provide supporting evidence. State a willingness to cooperate in finding a solution and then match behaviors to words. Persist in the pursuit of a solution (Ruthman, 2008). See Table 3-12 for a checklist for enhancing your ability to work with your boss. You may find it helpful to use a personal process recording to examine and improve your communications. See Table 3-13.

TABLE 3-12

HOW TO IMPROVE YOUR ABILITY TO WORK WITH YOUR BOSS

Know your boss's
- Goals and objectives
- Pressures
- Strengths, weaknesses, and blind spots
- Working style

Understand your own
- Objectives
- Pressures
- Strengths, weaknesses, and blind spots
- Working style
- Predisposition toward dependence on authority figures

Develop a relationship with your boss that
- Meets both your objectives and styles
- Keeps your boss informed
- Is based on dependability and honesty
- Selectively uses your boss's time and resources

Adapted from *Managing your boss,* by J. J. Gabarro and J. P. Kotter, Harvard Business Review, May–June, 1993, 150–157.

TABLE 3-13
PROCESS RECORDING EXCERPT

Interaction		Communication Technique Used	Evaluation
Nurse preceptor:	What has been going on with you this week?	Broad Opening	Permits nurse to begin with what is important at the moment
Nurse 2:	I have been thinking a lot about my job. I feel like I don't delegate care the way that I should.		
Nurse preceptor:	You are not delegating care well enough?	Restating	Provides chance for nurse 2 to expand on thoughts
Nurse 2:	No. I think that I should be doing better.		
Nurse preceptor:	So, you think you should be doing better?	Reflection	Returns nurse 2 to feelings. Nurse 2 is then able to talk about past experiences
Nurse 2:	Yes, I find it hard to tell someone else what to do. I worry that my patients won't get good care if I don't learn delegation, as I can't do all the nursing care myself. I need the help of others.		
Nurse preceptor:	Others?	Clarification	Allows nurse preceptor to seek information, yet encourages nurse 2 to go on
Nurse 2:	Yes, I need some more help to get better at delegation.		
Nurse preceptor:	OK, let's work together.		

EVIDENCE FROM THE LITERATURE

Citation: Tulgan, B. (2007, September). It's okay to be boss—be a great one! *Nursing Management, 38*(9), 20–24.

Discussion: The author states that health care professionals need leaders who are willing and able to put in the time and effort to practice the art of real empowerment—guidance, direction, and support. The author advocates hands-on management with the following eight steps.

1. Get in the habit of managing every day. Set aside time to meet with your staff. The goal is to make these one-on-one sessions routine, brief, straight, and simple.
2. Learn to talk like a performance coach. Develop a way of talking that is both demanding and supportive, disciplined and patient. Be sure to tune in to the individual you're coaching; focus on specific instances of individual performance; describe the employee's performance honestly and vividly; develop concrete next steps.
3. Take it one person at a time. Continually ask yourself these key questions:
   a. Who is this person at work?
   b. Why do I need to manage this person?
   c. What do I need to talk about with this person?
   d. How should I talk with this person?
   e. Where should I talk with this person?
   f. When should I talk with this person?
4. Make accountability a real process. Employees must trust and believe that this is a fair and accurate process. Be sure to
   a. Focus on concrete actions within the direct control of the employee.
   b. Hold people accountable.
   c. Raise your standards.
   d. Separate your role as the boss from your personal relationships. If your authority is limited, use influence.
5. Clarify what to do and how to do it. Spell out your expectations and convert them into standard operating procedures—and then require employees to follow those procedures precisely.
6. Follow performance every step of the way. You need to be able to reference an ongoing written record of exactly what expectations, goals, deadlines, and requirements were established and met. Monitor, measure, and document performance—good, bad, and average—with every employee, every step of the way.
7. Solve small problems before they turn into big problems. Have regular management conversations with a strong goal focus. This will give you a natural venue in which to provide regular evaluation and feedback. Remember that addressing one small problem after another is what ongoing continuous performance improvement actually looks like.

(continues)

Evidence from the Literature *(continued)*

8. Based on their performance and your goals, do more for some employees and less for others. Give every person the chance to meet the basic expectations of his or her job and then the chance to go above and beyond—and to be rewarded accordingly. Be generous and flexible. Expand your repertoire of rewards and start using every resource you have to drive performance. Make a point of making special deals and small accommodations in exchange for extra performance.

Implications for Practice: The author suggests that you should be the boss who says, "Great news, I'm the boss! I consider that a sacred responsibility. I'm going to set you up for success every step of the way. I'm going to help you plan. I'm going to work with you to clarify goals, guidelines, and specifications. I'm going to help you find the shortcuts, avoid the pitfalls, and follow the best practices. Count on me. When you need something, I'm going to help you find it. When you want something, I'm going to help you earn it." Work to be this kind of boss.

COMMUNICATING WITH CO-WORKERS

Nurses work directly or indirectly with a wide variety of people. One of the challenges in working in health care is the interdisciplinary focus that revolves around patient care delivery. Sovie (1992) discusses the need for high-quality teams in health care that have a specific purpose and that contribute to the organization's overall outcomes performance. A registered nurse is directly responsible for the care of the patient, and that care includes ensuring that the correct medical and nursing orders are carried out. For example, an RN must make sure that the correct medication dosage was transcribed, that the NAP documented the correct intake and output accurately for the shift, that the LPN/LVN completed the ordered treatments, that the discharge planning was coordinated with the social worker and case manager, that the pharmacist distributed the medications, that the family understands how to dress the patient's wound, and finally, that the patient understands the discharge instructions. Nurses depend on their co-workers in many ways to collectively provide quality patient care. Nowhere is this more important than in the acute care setting, where nursing services are nonstop around the clock.

An excellent guide for directing communication with co-workers is to treat them with respect, as you would want to be treated. As a nurse who will be responsible for overseeing others' work, a valuable perspective to maintain is that all members of the team are important to successfully realize quality patient care. Communication between nurses and co-workers will usually involve delegating. Offering positive feedback such as, "I appreciate the way you interacted with Mr. T. to get him to ambulate twice this shift" goes a long way toward team building, and it improves co-workers' sense of worth. Nurses also have an opportunity to act as teachers to co-workers. In a hospital setting, nurses often teach by example. Demonstrating the desired behavior allows co-workers to copy the behavior. It is important to allow time for return demonstrations to evaluate that the co-workers have learned the intended skill. For example, as the nurse, you may demonstrate how to position a patient with special needs, encouraging a co-worker to assist and ask questions. The next time repositioning is indicated, accompany the co-worker and observe his or her ability to successfully complete the task. Offer constructive feedback. Be patient. Remember your own learning curves when mastering new skills and behaviors and allow those you supervise the opportunity to grow. Be open to the possibility that co-workers, particularly those with experience, may have a few pearls of wisdom to share with you as well (Ruthman, 2008). See Tables 3-14 and 3-15.

TABLE 3-14
BUILDING A SUCCESSFUL TEAM

Davis, Hellervik, Sheard, Skube, and Gebelein (1996) offer the following suggestions for building a successful team:
- Value the contributions of all team members: All members are critical to the success of the team regardless of their position on the team.
- Encourage interaction among group members: Know when verbal and nonverbal behavior is appropriate and inappropriate, and keep the flow of communication going.
- Discourage "we versus they" thinking: Build teamwork that encourages inter-team participation and relationships.
- Involve others in shaping plans and decisions: Involving the total team in problem solving and decision making will strengthen any suggested changes made by the team because the entire team is able to support the decisions.
- Acknowledge and celebrate team accomplishments: Publicly and frequently acknowledge positive contributions by team members, and keep the team members abreast of the positive changes they are actively involved in making.
- Evaluate your effectiveness as a team member: Being an effective team leader includes being an effective team member. Are you carrying your weight, or are you expecting others to carry out your directives?

TABLE 3-15
SELECTED TIPS ON CIVILITY

• Smile.	• Keep your voice low in public places.
• Give praise.	
• Admit when you are wrong.	• Do not ridicule, humiliate, or demean others.
• Let others be kind to you.	
	• Show consideration.

COMMUNICATING WITH HEALTH CARE PRACTITIONERS

Communicating with nursing and health care providers need not be intimidating or stressful. The nurse's goal is to strive for collaboration, keeping the patient goal central to the discussion. Collaboration allows all parties to be satisfied. It improves quality and is an attribute of magnet hospitals (Arford, 2005). It involves seeking creative, integrative solutions while also working through emotions. To communicate effectively with a practitioner, the nurse presents information in a straightforward manner, clearly delineating the problem, supported by pertinent evidence. This is especially important when reporting changes in patient conditions. Nurses are responsible for knowing classic symptoms of conditions, orally apprising the practitioner of changes, and recording all observations in the chart. It is important that the nurse remain calm and objective even if the practitioner does not cooperate. Calfee (1998) offers suggestions for handling telephone miscommunications. For example, if a practitioner hangs up, document that the call was terminated and fill out an incident report. If the practitioner gives an inappropriate answer or gives no orders, for example, for a patient complaint of pain, document the call, the information relayed, and the fact that no orders were given. In addition, document any other steps that were taken to resolve the problems, for example, notifying the nursing supervisor. If a practitioner cannot be reached, first follow the institution's procedure for getting the patient treated and then document the actions taken.

Show respect and consideration for the health care providers that you work with, but don't be a doormat. Give due respect and expect the same from them. Present information in a straightforward manner, clearly delineating the problem and offering pertinent evidence. See Table 3-16 for a tool to organize patient information prior to calling another practitioner or doctor for assistance.

EVIDENCE FROM THE LITERATURE

Citation: Haig, K. M., Sutton, S., & Whittington, J. (2006). The SBARR technique: Improves communication, enhances patient safety. *Joint Commission's Perspectives on Patient Safety, 5*(2), 1–2.

Discussion: Communication failures are the root cause of nearly two-thirds of sentinel events in hospitals. This is due, in part, because nursing and medical practitioners and nurses are trained to communicate differently. The SBAR (Situation, Background, Assessment, Recommendation) technique is designed to improve communication between these health care personnel:

- *Situation:* What is going on with the patient? Identify self, unit, patient, and room number. Briefly state the problem, when it started, and its severity.
- *Background:* Provide background information related to the situation, as needed. Be aware of patient's admitting diagnosis, date of admission, current medications, allergies, IV fluids, most recent vital signs, lab results with date and time each was performed, other clinical information, and patient code status. The practitioner may ask you for these when you call.
- *Assessment:* What is your assessment? Do you think the patient's condition is deteriorating? Do you think the patient needs medication?
- *Recommendation:* What is your recommendation or what do you want? Know what you want from the practitioner before you call. Don't hang up without communicating this to the practitioner and assuring that your patient's needs are met, e.g., patient needs to be admitted, patient needs to be seen, order needs to be changed, or medication needs to be added.
- *Response:* Document response of practitioner.

Implications for Practice: Nursing and medical practitioners who use the SBARR technique will improve their communications. Patients will be the beneficiaries.

TABLE 3-16

SBARR TOOL TO ORGANIZE INFORMATION FOR CALLING ANOTHER NURSING OR MEDICAL PRACTITIONER FOR ASSISTANCE

Situation:
Identify date and time of call.
Identify self, unit, patient, room number, and admitting diagnosis.
State the problem: what it is, when it started, and the severity of it.

(continues)

Table 3-16 *(continued)*

Background:
Review background information related to the situation. Identify current medications, allergies, IV fluids, vital signs, level of consciousness, urine output, status of airway, breathing, circulation, pain level, pulse oximeter, cardiac rhythm, lab results, patient code status, and other clinical information.

Assessment:
What is your assessment of the patient? Is the patient's problem severe? Is his or her condition deteriorating? Does the patient need medication?

Recommendation:
What is needed from the practitioner? Know what you want from the practitioner before you call. Don't hang up without communicating this to the practitioner and assuring that your patient's needs are met, for example, patient needs to be admitted, patient needs to be seen, patient needs medication, and so on.

Response:
Document response of practitioner. Document all calls to practitioner and messages left. Notify supervisor when needed for follow-up.

Adapted from *SBARR: A shared mental model for improving communication between clinicians* by K. M. Haig, S. Sutton, and J. Whittington, 2006.

REAL WORLD INTERVIEW

As an emergency medicine physician, I am frequently interfacing with nurses during life-threatening medical scenarios. Whether it is an acute myocardial infarction or respiratory failure or even a very sick child, the dialogue is standard. There is a set tone of urgency on both our parts, and we get straight to work with little discussion. I think when we work as a team, we are like a well-oiled machine. The nurse anticipates my needs and I hers or his, and we follow our protocols. The absolute focus is on the patient, and getting him or her out of immediate danger. That is what the emergency department does best. We "stabilize" the patient's acute life-threatening event. The rapport between MD and RN is built from an understanding of mutual competency. I know my nurses in the ED and they know me. I could not save lives day in and day out without this teamwork mentality.

Dr. Elizabeth Horvath, DO
Crystal Lake, Illinois

If the practitioner gives you a verbal or telephone order, be sure to repeat the order back to the practitioner and document after the written order, Telephone Order Repeated Back (TORB) or Verbal Order Repeated Back (VORB).

In all cases, nurses must remember that since the RN owes a duty directly to the patient, blindly relying on another nursing or medical practitioner's judgment is not permissible.

EVIDENCE FROM THE LITERATURE

Citation: Sirota, T. (2008, July). Nurse/Physician relationships: Survey report. *Nursing, 38*(7), 28–31.

Discussion: More than half of respondents to this survey of nurses—57%—say they're generally satisfied with their professional relations with physicians; a significant minority, 43%, reports dissatisfaction. Respondents' comments indicate that they perceive several factors to be at play here:
- Male physicians' perceptions of traditional gender and cultural roles
- Physicians' arrogance and feelings of superiority
- Nurses' feelings of inferiority
- Hospital culture or policy reinforcing a subordinate role for nurses

Important ways to improve nurse/physician overall collaboration identified in the article include workplace empowerment for nurses, nurse/physician rounds, team meetings, collaborative educational programs, and collaborative membership on hospital committees (Sirota, 2008).

The article states that the bottom line is that nurses aren't expendable. Given the current nursing shortage, the climate is ripe for nurses to speak up as a group and let facility administrators know that they need to pay attention to nurses' legitimate concerns about nurse/physician collaboration, and then correct deficiencies.

Perhaps most importantly, improving relationships between nurses and physicians will benefit both professional groups by improving job satisfaction and productivity, and will benefit patients by enhancing their overall safety, welfare, and clinical progress. This can be accomplished by promoting greater nurse/physician professional respect, improving communication and collaboration, educating physicians about nursing roles and skills, and addressing physician misconduct (Rosenstein, Russell, & Lauve, 2002).

Implications for Practice: Nursing and medical practitioner communication has improved since the 1991 survey. Good communication by all members of the health care team affects patient safety and must be facilitated by nursing, medical, and hospital team members to build an environment for patient safety.

CREW RESOURCE MANAGEMENT

Patient care, like other technically complex and high-risk fields, is an interdependent process carried out by teams of individuals with advanced technical training who have varying roles and decision-making responsibilities. While technical training assures proficiency at specific tasks, it does not address the potential for errors created by communication and decision making in dynamic environments. Experts in aviation have developed safety training focused on effective team management, known as Crew Resource Management (CRM). Improvements in the safety record of commercial aviation may be due, in part, to this training (Helmreich, 2000). Over the past 20 years, lessons from aviation's approach to team training have been applied to patient safety, notably in the intensive care unit (ICU) (Shortell et al., 1994) and anesthesia training (Howard, Gaba, Fish, Yang, & Sarnquist, 1992). CRM training encompasses a wide range of knowledge, skills, and attitudes including communicating assertively, being situationally aware, and using problem solving, decision making, and teamwork. See Table 3-17.

"Assertive behavior" is the willingness to actively participate, state, and maintain a position, until convinced by the facts that other options are better. It requires initiative and the courage to act. "Situational awareness" refers to the degree of accuracy by which one's perception of his or her current environment mirrors reality. Factors that reduce situational awareness include insufficient communication, fatigue/stress, task overload, task underload, group mindset, "press on regardless" philosophy, and degraded operating conditions.

CRM fosters a climate or culture in which the freedom to respectfully question authority is encouraged. However, the primary goal of CRM is not enhanced communication, but enhanced situational awareness. It recognizes

TABLE 3-17
BEHAVIORS

Passive	Assertive	Aggressive
Overly courteous	Actively involved	Dominates
"Beats around the bush"	Ready to take action	Intimidates
Avoids conflicts	Provides useful information	Acts abusively or hostilely
"Along for the ride"	Makes suggestions, speaks up	Attacks

Compiled with info from LISTCrew Resource Management (CRM) Training: Guidance For Flight Crew, CRM Instructors (CRMIS) and CRM Instructor-Examiners (CRMIES). (2006). Accessed March 14, 2010, from http://www.globalaviation.com/_downloads/cap737.pdf

that a discrepancy between what is happening and what should be happening is often the first indicator that an error is occurring. This is a delicate subject for many organizations, especially ones with traditional hierarchies like those seen in health care. Appropriate communication techniques must be taught to all nursing and medical practitioners so they understand that the questioning of authority need not be threatening, and so that all understand the correct way to question orders.

A CRM expert named Todd Bishop developed a five-step assertive statement process that encompasses inquiry and advocacy steps. The five steps are
- Opening or attention getter: Address the individual. "Dr. Karen" or "Michelle," or whatever name or title will get the person's attention.
- State your concern: State what you see in a direct manner while owning your emotions about it. "Mr. Jones has a pulse of 160."
- State the problem as you see it: "Mr. Jones is going into ventricular tachycardia."
- State a solution: "Mr. Jones needs an antiarrhythmic medication."
- Obtain agreement (or buy-in): "Do you want to order an antiarrhythmic medication?"

These are difficult but important skills to master, as they require a change in interpersonal dynamics and organizational culture.

Adapted from Crew Resource Management (International Association of Fire Chiefs, 2003).

CASE STUDY 3-2

Your nurse manager has assigned you as the new member of the task force on patient falls. This task force has been meeting for almost a year without making much progress. In coming to your first meeting, you note that there are several challenging personalities on the team and wonder if they will ever be able to work together effectively.

Jamie is a new graduate nurse and volunteers for everything. Angela likes details, often asking everyone to repeat what they said so that she can get more information on the topic. Samantha is the passive one and looks annoyed at having to be there. You noticed she was doing some of her patient charting while in the meeting. Anabelle attempts to keep the team on track, but with her soft-spoken voice, she is not well heard. Finally, no matter what anyone says, Beth is critical and comes up with a reason why something will not work.

Would the Myers-Briggs Type Indicator give you any more information about the members of this team?

It would be interesting to use the MBTI and have each member of the team identify his or her personal MBTI type. Then the team members can compare the different types represented in the group. See the online test in the Web Exercises.

REVIEW QUESTIONS

1. The nurse has become incredibly busy with discharging two patients and expecting a new patient any second. The following is a list of tasks that need to be completed right away. What task can the nurse delegate to a NAP to help out with managing the nurse's time?
   A. Transport a patient to X-ray on a cardiac monitor.
   B. Sit with a patient who was recently diagnosed with Crohn's disease who is crying.
   C. Remove sutures from an incision and drainage (I&D) of the left wrist.
   D. Provide tracheostomy care.

2. An LPN is assigned to pass medications on seven patients. Several hours later one of the patients complained to the RN that he had not received his medication. How will the nurse handle this situation to ensure this task was completed based on the Five Rights of Delegation?
   A. Disregard the patient's complaint and give the medication.
   B. Discuss with the LPN the recent complaint by the patient.
   C. Follow the LPN during the next medication administration.
   D. Ask all the patients if they have received their medications.

3. The nurse delegated to the nursing assistant to turn a particular patient. After an hour had gone by, the nurse asked the nursing assistant if the patient had been turned. The nursing assistant replied "No." What should the nurse have done to ensure the task was completed?
   A. Assist the NAP when turning the patient.
   B. Not delegate this inappropriate task to a NAP.
   C. Explain the procedure to the nursing assistant.
   D. Inform the NAP of the time frame in which the task was to be completed.

4. The nurse asks a NAP who works on the unit who is also a nursing student if the student wants to flush an IV site after the antibiotic infuses. Of course the answer is yes, because the NAP wants to know as much or even more than their fellow students and would hope for more opportunities. Is it okay for a nursing student to complete this delegated task?
   A. Yes, in a student role, but not as a NAP
   B. Yes, as long as the student has been taught how to flush an IV site
   C. No, students or NAP are never allowed to flush an IV site in any situation
   D. Yes, if the nurse verifies that the NAP can perform the procedure

5. A new graduate nurse asks the charge nurse, "How do I know what I can and cannot delegate?" What is the best reply for the charge nurse?
   A. "You will not be delegating, only the charge nurse delegates, so there is nothing to worry about."
   B. "Delegation takes time and practice to learn what you can and cannot do."
   C. "Every state has standards, laws, and guidelines for delegation to guide you."
   D. "If you follow the Five Rights of medication administration you should be fine."

6. An RN asks the NAP to take a set of vital signs on a patient who has just had an arterial venous shunt placement. The RN reminds the NAP not to take the blood pressure (BP) on the operative side. An hour later, the RN finds the deflated blood pressure cuff on the operative arm of the patient. The NAP has done this before and has been counseled about it. What should the RN do first?
   A. Assess the patient's condition.
   B. Avoid asking this NAP to take BPs in the future.
   C. Discuss the situation with the NAP and the supervisor.
   D. Find the NAP and review the importance of taking the blood pressure on the non-operative side.

7. Why must nurses be concerned about barriers to communication?
   A. Because they enhance interactions
   B. So that they can use them when communicating
   C. Nurses don't need to be concerned
   D. So that they can overcome them

8. A health care provider walks into a patient's room as the nurse is administering medications correctly through the G-tube (gastric feeding tube). The health care provider says to the nurse, "obviously you have never done that before—give me the syringe and let me administer the medications." What is the best way for the nurse to respond?
   A. "I have administered medications through a G-tube before—do you see a problem with my technique?"
   B. "Why do you think I have never done this before?"
   C. "Why don't we discuss this matter in the hallway?"
   D. "I know you were once a nurse, but now you are a practitioner and you are not allowed to perform these tasks."

APPLY YOUR SKILLS

1. The charge nurse apologizes as she informs you that your assignment includes the "problem NAP" on the unit. What communication skills will you use to enhance communication with this NAP? How will you avoid barriers in communication with this NAP?

2. You found out that you passed your NCLEX last month. When you report for your evening shift, you discover you are assigned to be the team leader. What communication skills will you use to communicate with the other nursing and health care providers?

3. Check out this site for the MBTI (www.personalitypathways.com.) Decide what MBTI type you are, and ask a friend or colleague to identify what type they think you are. It is always informative to discover if you see yourself the way that others see you.

4. Mary is feeling more confident that she has the knowledge level she needs to safely care for her patients. She would like to improve her ability to work with and delegate to the NAP on her unit. How can she proceed? How can Mary use the four Cs of communication discussed in Table 3-1 to delegate effectively?

5. Angela, an RN, has been working on the unit for almost a year now and is working as a preceptor to Josie, a new graduate nurse. Angela remembers what it was like to be a novice and is trying to help Josie adapt to her new role. Angela recalls that it took her a long time to perform her duties when she first started, and she tells Josie this fact.

   Angela also notes that her skills increased as she assumed more personal responsibility for learning new skills and as she became comfortable with both the policies and procedures of the unit and with her own and her staff's job descriptions. Angela tells Josie to expect it to take a while to become skilled in her role. Angela suggests that Josie use Table 3-4 to guide her in her role preparation. How can you use Table 3-4 to take personal responsibility for developing your professional nursing role?

EXPLORING THE WEB

1. Search for information about the MBTI tool at:
   www.typelogic.com
   www.keirsey.com
   www.humanmetrics.com

2. Visit the Web site of The Joint Commission to review annual National Patient Safety Goals:
   www.jointcommission.org

3. Go to www.allnurses.com to discuss communication issues and other pertinent issues associated with nursing.
4. Visit www.virtualnurse.com as an excellent reference for nursing information, from continuing education courses to research related to communication and other nursing topics.
5. The University of Minnesota Center for Gerontological Nursing has compiled a list of Web sites for their Center. Search for the communication resources to use when working with elderly patients at www.nursing.umn.edu
6. Visit these Web sites to discover some nursing journals online:
www.nursingcenter.com
www.medscape.com
www.nursingmanagement.com
7. Research www.nsna.org as a guide to education and careers in nursing, which includes the most comprehensive directory of nursing schools with full school profiles, as well as detailed nursing questions and answers.
8. Visit this University of Michigan site for time management tips:
www.umich.edu
Search for stress manager.

REFERENCES

American Nurses Association. (2003). *Nursing social policy statement* (2nd ed.). Washington, DC: American Nurses Publishing.

American Nurses Association. (2008). *Professional Role Competence.* Accessed March 14, 2010, from www.nursingworld.org/NursingPractice

Andrews, L. B., Stocking, C. T., Krizek, T., Gottlieb, L., Krizek, C., Vargish, T., et al. (1997, Febuary). An alternative strategy for studying adverse events in medical care. *Lancet, 349,* 309–313.

Arford, P. H. (2005). Nurse-physician communication: An organizational accountability. *Nursing Economics, 23*(2), 72–77.

Baggs, J. G., Ryan, S. A., Phelps, C. E., Richeson, J. F., & Johnson, J. E. (1992). The association between interdisciplinary collaboration and patient outcomes in a medical intensive care unit. *Heart and Lung, 21*(1), 18–24.

Baker, C., Beglinger, J., King, S., Salyards, M., & Thompson, A. (2000). Transforming negative work cultures. *JONA, 30*(7/8), 357–363.

Bartol, K., & Martin, D. (1998). *Management* (3rd ed.). Boston, MA: McGraw-Hill.

Calfee, B. E. (1998). Making calls to the physician. *Nursing, 28*(10), 17.

Chatman, J., & O'Reilly, C. (2004). Asymmetric effects of work group demographics on men's and women's responses to work group composition. *Academy of Management Journal, 47*(2), 193–208.

Davis, B. L., Hellervik, L. W., Sheard, J. L., Gebelein, S. H., & Skube, C. J. (1996). *Successful manager's handbook.* Minneapolis, MN: Personnel Decisions Pub.

Deber, R. B., & Leatt, P. (1986). The multidisciplinary renal team: Who makes the decisions? *Health Matrix, 4*(3), 3–9.

DuBrin, A. J. (2000). *The active manager.* United Kingdom: South-Western Pub.

Ellis, A. (2002). *Anger: How to live with and without it.* New York, NY: Kensington Publishing Corporation.

Frisch, N. C., & Frisch, L. E. (2011). *Psychiatric mental health nursing* (4th ed.). Clifton Park, NY: Delmar Cengage Learning.

Gabarro, J. J., & Kotter, J. P. (1993, May–June). Managing your boss. *Harvard business review, 71*(3), 150–157.

Giger, J. N., & Davidhizar, R. E. (2008). *Transcultural nursing* (5th ed.). Baltimore, MD: Mosby.

Gittell, J. H., Fairfield, K. M., Bierbaum, G., Head, W., Jackson, R., Kelly, M., et al. (2000). Impact of relational coordination of quality of care, postoperative pain and functioning, and length of stay: A nine-hospital study of surgical patients. *Medical Care, 38*(8), 807–819.

Gray, J. (2001). *Mars and Venus in the workplace: A practical guide for improving communication & getting results at work.* New York, NY: Harper Collins.

Haig, K. M., Sutton, S., & Whittington, J. (2006). The SBARR technique: Improves communication, enhances patient safety. *Joint Commission's Perspectives on Patient Safety, 5*(2), 1–2.

Helmreich, R. L. (2000, March 18). On error management: Lessons from aviation. *British Medical Journal, 320*(7237), 781–785.

Howard, S. K., Gaba, D. M., Fish, K. J., Yang, G., & Sarnquist, F. H. (1992, September) Anesthesia crisis resource management training: Teaching anesthesiologists to handle critical incidents. *Aviation, Space, and Environmental Medicine, 63*(9), 763–770.

Institute of Medicine. (2003). *Keeping patients safe: Transforming the environment of nurses.* Washington, DC: National Academics Press.

International Association of Fire Chiefs. (2003). Crew Resource Management: A Positive Change for the Fire Service. Fairfax, VA: Author.

Isabel, B. M., & Myers, P. B. (1995). *Gifts differing.* Palo Alto, CA: Davies-Black.

Janis, L. (1972). *Victims of groupthink.* Boston, MA: Houghton Mifflin.

Keirsey, D., & Bates, M. (1978). *Please understand me: Character and temperament types.* Del Mar, CA: Prometheus Nemesis Books.

Kelly, P. (2010). Patient teaching. In P. Kelly (Ed.), *Essentials of Nursing leadership & management* (2nd ed.) (pp. 300–325). Clifton Park, NY: Delmar Cengage Learning.

Kinney, M., & Hurst, J. (1979). *Group process in education.* Lexington, MA: Ginn Customs.

Knaus, W. A., Draper, E. A., Wagner, D. P., & Zimmerman, J. E. (1986). An evaluation of outcome from intensive care in major medical centers. *Annals of Internal Medicine, 104*(3), 410–418.

Longo, J., & Sherman, R. O. (2007, March). Leveling horizontal violence. *Nursing Management, 38*(3), 34–37.

Mitchell, P., & Grippando, G. (1994). *Nursing perspectives and issues.* Albany, NY: Delmar Publishers.

Munoz, C., & Luckmann, J. (2005). *Transcultural communication in nursing* (2nd ed.). Clifton Park, NY: Delmar Cengage Learning.

Needleman, J., Buerhaus, P., Mattke, S., Stewart, M., & Zelevinsky, K. (2002). Nurse-staffing levels and the quality of care in hospitals. *New England Journal of Medicine, 346*(22), 1715–1722.

Northouse, P. G., & Northouse, L. L. (1997). *Health communication: Strategies for health professionals* (3rd ed.). Norwalk, CT: Appleton and Lange.

Owens, D. A., Mannic, E. A., & Neale, M. A. (1998). Strategic formation of groups: Issues in task performance and team member selection. In D. H. Gruenfeld (Ed.), *Research on managing groups and teams* (pp. 149–165). Stanford, CT: MAI Press.

Polifko-Harris, K. (2008). Effective team building. In P. L. Kelly (Ed.), *Nursing leadership & management* (2nd ed.). Clifton Park, NY: Delmar Cengage Learning.

Rosenstein, A. H., Russell, H., & Lauve, R. (2002, November–December). Disruptive physician behavior contributes to nursing shortage: Study links bad behavior by doctors to nurses leaving the profession. *Physician Executive, 28*(6), 8–11.

Ruthman, J. (2008). Personal and interdisciplinary communication. In P. L. Kelly (Ed.), *Nursing leadership & management* (2nd ed.). Clifton Park, NY: Delmar Cengage Learning.

Schmitt, M. H. (2001). Collaboration improves the quality of care: Methodological challenges and evidence from health care research. *Journal of Interprofessional Care, 15*, 47–66.

Scott, W. G. (1967). *Organization Theory.* Homewood, IL: Irwin.

Shi, L., & Singh, D. A. (2001). *Delivering health care in America* (2nd ed.). Aspen, CO: Aspen Publishers.

Shortell, S. M., & Kaluzny, A. D. (2006). *Health Care Management.* Clifton Park, NY: Delmar Cengage Learning.

Shortell, S. M., Zimmerman, J. E., Rousseau, D. M., Gillies, R. R., Wagner, D. P., Draper, E. A., et al. (1994). The performance of intensive care units: Does good management make a difference? *Medical Care, 32*(5), 508–525.

Sirota, T. (2008, July). Nurse/Physician relationships: Survey report. *Nursing, 38*(7), 28–31.

Sovie, M. (1992). Care and service teams: A new imperative. *Nursing Economic, 10*(2), 94–100.

Topping, S., Norton, T., & Scafidi, B. (2003). Coordination of services: The use of multidisciplinary interagency teams. In S. Dopson and A. L. Mark (Eds.), *Leading Health Care Organizations* (pp. 100–112). New York, NY: Palgrave Macmillan.

Tulgan, B. (2007, September). It's okay to be the boss—be a great one! *Nursing Management, 38*(9), 18–24.

Wiseman, R. (2004). *The luck factor: The four essential principles.* New York, NY: Miramax.

Young, G. J., Charns, M. P., Daley, J., Forbes, M. G., Henderson, W., & Khuri, S. F. (1997). Best practices for managing surgical services: The role of coordination. *Health Care Management Review, 22*(4), 72–81.

Young, G. J., Charns, M. P., Desai, K., Khuri, S. F., Forbes, M. G., Henderson, W., et al. (1998, December). Patterns of coordination and clinical outcomes: A study of surgical services. *Health Services Research, 33*(5, Pt. 1),1211–1236.

Zerwekh, J., & Claborn, J. (2009). *Nursing today: Transition and trends* (6th ed.). St. Louis, MO: Saunders.

SUGGESTED READINGS

Cardillo, D. W. (2001). *Your first year as a nurse.* Roseville, CA: Prima.

Colón-Emeric, C. S. (2006). Patterns of medical and nursing staff communication in nursing homes: Implications and insights from complexity science. *Qualitative Health Research, 16*(2), 173–188.

Lachman, V. D. (2008). Making ethical choices: Weighing obligations and virtues. *Nursing 2008, 38*(10), 42–46.

Manojlovich, M. (2005). Linking the practice environment to nurses' job satisfaction through nurse-physician communication. *Journal of Nursing Scholarship, 37*(4), 367–373.

Urrabazo-Kane, C. (2009). Management's role in shaping organizational culture. *Journal of Nursing Management, 14*(3), 188–194.

CHAPTER 4

Time Management, Setting Priorities, and Making Assignments

Patricia Kelly, Patsy L. Maloney, Maureen T. Marthaler

Time is the coin of your life. It is the only coin you have, and only you can determine how it will be spent.
—Carol
  Sandberg

OBJECTIVES

Upon completion of this chapter, the reader should be able to:

1. Discuss general time management techniques.

2. Analyze the use of professional nursing and personal time.

3. Review time wasters.

4. Discuss behaviors of perfectionists versus pursuers of excellence.

5. Discuss effective use of available time.

6. Describe setting priorities for safe patient care.

7. Discuss shift handoff report.

8. Review a shift action plan.

9. Practice making assignments.

Lateisha has just completed her medical-surgical orientation as a new graduate registered nurse. This evening is her first solo shift. But she is not really alone. Lateisha, Mary, the charge nurse, and one nursing assistive personnel (NAP) are responsible for eight patients in this section of the unit. Currently there are seven patients, and a new admission is on the way. The patient from the recovery room has just returned from gall bladder surgery, the dinner trays are arriving, and Lateisha has medications to pass. Just as the dinner trays arrive, the daughter of Mrs. Glusak runs out to Lateisha and states that her mom seems more confused and is incontinent. Her mother has just pulled out her IV, and it is leaking on the floor.

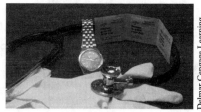

Delmar Cengage Learning

What would you do first if you were Lateisha?

How can Lateisha manage her time and set priorities?

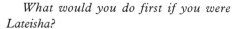

Many people become nurses out of idealism. They want to help others. Unfortunately, most new graduates find it impossible to meet all, or even most, of their patients' needs. Needs tend to be unlimited while time is limited. In addition to direct patient care responsibilities, there are shift responsibilities, charting, doctor's orders to be transcribed or checked, medications to be administered, and patient reports to be given.

New graduates often go home feeling totally inadequate. They wake up remembering what they did not accomplish. One young nurse, with tears in her eyes, shared that once, when she answered a call late in her shift, the patient requested a pain medication. She went to the medication room to get the medication but was interrupted by an emergency situation. When she arrived home, she was so exhausted that she fell asleep rapidly, only to awaken with the realization that she had not returned with her patient's medication. Her guilt was tremendous. She had gone into nursing to relieve pain, not to ignore it.

Using time management skills and setting priorities allow the new nurse to prioritize care, decide on outcomes, and perform or delegate the most important interventions first. Time management skills are not just important for nurses on the job. It is important for their personal lives as well. Time management allows nurses to make time for fun, friends, exercise, and professional development (Maloney, 2008). This chapter discusses general time management tips and the setting of priorities, and also illustrates a way to analyze professional and personal time. It considers behaviors of perfectionists versus pursuers of excellence and discusses shift handoff reports, patient rounds, and how to make assignments.

GENERAL TIME MANAGEMENT TECHNIQUES

Time management has been defined as "a set of related common-sense skills that helps people use their time in the most effective and productive way possible" (Mind Tools, 1999–2006). In other words, time management allows people to achieve more with the available time they have. Time management requires self-examination of what pursuits are really important, analysis of how time is currently being used, and assessment of the distractions that have been siphoning time from more important pursuits.

Time management requires a shift from being busy to getting things done, a shift from focusing on the process of work to focusing on achieving a good work outcome. A busy frenzy is often reinforced with sympathy and assistance from others. Too often this frenzied behavior is accomplishing very little, because it is not directed at the right outcome. There is a simple principle, the **Pareto Principle**, which states that 20% of focused effort results in 80% of desired outcomes or results, or conversely that 80% of unfocused effort results in 20% of results (Pareto Principle, 2008). See Figure 4-1.

The Pareto Principle, named after Vilfredo Pareto, was invoked by the Total Quality Management (TQM) movement and J. M. Juran, and is now reemerging as a strategy for balancing life and work through prioritization of effort. It is important to analyze how your time is being used to manage available time and achieve desired outcomes.

If good time management achieves desired outcomes, why do so many people move at a crazy, hurried pace? There are several possible explanations for this. They do not know about time management, they think they do not have time to plan, they do not want to stop to plan, or they love crises (Mind Tools, 1999–2006).

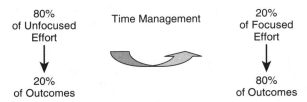

80% of Unfocused Effort	Time Management	20% of Focused Effort
↓		↓
20% of Outcomes		80% of Outcomes

Figure 4-1 The Pareto Principle. (Delmar Cengage Learning.)

KEEP YOUR PATIENTS SAFE 4-1

When you ask overworked nurses why they did not plan their shift, they often say that they did not have time. Do you think they really did not have time? Jumping into your work without a plan is like starting a journey without looking at a map. How much time would you waste if you just started driving? Think about this the next time you work. What outcomes do you want to achieve? What is your plan for achieving these outcomes?

OUTCOME ORIENTATION

With the Pareto Principle in mind, it is important to recognize that more is achieved through an outcome orientation than through an emphasis on the process of task completion. Long-term goals must be determined. It is best to break long-term goals down into achievable outcomes that are the steps toward long-term goals. Long-term goals cannot be achieved overnight. Long-term goals and outcomes should be written down in a planner or in a personal data assistant (PDA). Even though these goals are written, they should remain flexible. Flexibility should be built into any outcome orientation. There may come a time when the outcome may no longer be realistic or should be shifted to a more realistic goal as circumstances change (Reed & Pettigrew, 2006).

ANALYSIS OF NURSING TIME

Analysis of professional nursing time use is important in developing a plan to effectively use time. Nurses cannot possibly know how to better plan their time without knowing how they currently use time. When keeping track of time, it is important to consider the value of a nurse's time as well as the use of the time.

VALUE OF NURSING TIME

Nurses often undervalue their time. Consider salary and benefits. Benefits are frequently forgotten, but they comprise 15% to 30% of total cost per employee. If a nurse is making $26.00 an hour, benefits add $3.90 to $7.25 to the hourly cost of a nurse's time. The value of nursing time in this example, excluding what the organization is paying in worker's compensation and payroll taxes, is $29.90 to $33.25 per hour. In addition to this, the organization has also invested in nurse recruitment, orientation, and development.

Nursing time is a valuable commodity. Keeping this in mind will be invaluable when considering work that can be delegated to personnel who receive less compensation or when considering spending time on completing a task that does not support achieving an outcome (Maloney, 2008).

USE OF TIME

Numerous studies have shown how nurses use their time (Scharf, 1997; Upenieks, 1998; Urden & Roode, 1997; Doffield, Gordner, & Cathing-Paul, 2008).

Fitzgerald, Pearson, Walsh, Long, and Heinrich (2003) found a similar distribution to previous time studies: 34% of nursing time was spent giving direct care; 38% in indirect support activities including documentation, obtaining supplies, and professional communication; 8% on unit activities—cleaning and tidying; 7% on other activities, such as looking for other personnel, equipment, and professional reading; and 13% personal time for breaks, personal conversations, and reading (Figure 4-2).

Given such a distribution of nurses' time, shifting the use of time could have a major impact on outcomes. If non-nursing activities could be performed by non-nursing personnel instead of nurses, more time could be redirected toward essential nursing responsibilities.

How do you use your time? Memory and self-reporting of time are often unreliable. Nurses are often unaware of the time spent on personal activities as well as time spent working, socializing with colleagues, making and drinking coffee, snacking, and so on.

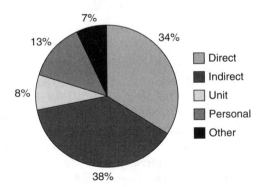

Figure 4-2 Use of nursing time. (Compiled with information from Patterns of nursing: A review of nursing in a large metropolitan hospital by M. Fitzgerald, A. Pearson, K. Walsh, L. Long, and N. Heinrich, 2003, *Journal of Clinical Nursing, 12*(3), 326–332.)

ACTIVITY LOG

An **activity log** is a time management tool that can assist the nurse in determining how both personal and professional time are used. The activity log (Table 4-1) should be used for several days.

Behavior should not be modified while keeping the activity log. The nurse should record every activity, from the beginning of the day until the end. Review of this log will illuminate good time use as well as time wasted. Analysis of the log will allow the separation of essential activities from activities that can be delegated to someone else (Grohar-Murray & DiCroce, 2003; Sullivan & Decker, 2004).

After completing the activity log, a nurse needs to consider all activities that have been completed, how much time each activity took, what outcome was achieved by performing the activities, and whether the activities could have been delegated to another. Notice your most energetic time of day. Activities that take focus and creativity should be scheduled at high-energy times and dull, repetitive tasks at low-energy times.

Use the activity log to examine relationships between eating patterns, rest patterns, and energy levels. If a nurse is tired and nonproductive after a large lunch, she or he should break the lunch down into several smaller snacks. Scheduling time for proper rest, exercise, and nutrition allows for quality time. When considering these questions, ask yourself, how would the Pareto Principle apply? Has 20% of focused effort resulted in 80% of outcome achievement? If the activities have not achieved the desired outcomes, the nurse needs to re-prioritize. Do this analysis with both your professional and personal time.

CREATING MORE TIME

There are several ways to create time. You can prioritize, or delegate work to others. Other ways include eliminating tasks that add no value and getting up earlier in the day. See Table 4-2 for strategies to avoid time wasters. Avoiding these time wasters will help you achieve excellence. You want to achieve excellence, not perfection! See Table 4-3.

When a person delegates a task, he or she cannot completely control when and how the task is completed. Initially, it may take more time to delegate a task to others than to do it oneself, but this investment of time should save time and energy in the future.

Getting up one hour earlier in the day can free up 365 hours, or approximately nine additional weeks a year. This extra time can be used to enrich life (Mind Tools, 1999–2006). This may be a good strategy for some people.

TABLE 4-1 *ACTIVITY LOG*				
Time	Name of activity-personal and professional (personal time, medication administration, vital signs, bed-making, patient transport, and so on)	Time required and feelings (energetic, bored, and so on)	Could be better done by someone else? Who? (LPN/LVN, nursing assistant, housekeeper, and so on)	Toward what outcome achievement? (increase in patient's functional status, prevention of complications, and so on)
0500	Treadmill	30 min – energetic	Keep for self	Fitness
0530	Shower and breakfast	45 min – energetic	Keep for self	Health
0615	Drive to work	10 min – alert	Keep for self	Get to work
0700	Shift handoff report	15 min – alert	Keep for self	Patient identification
0730	Patient rounds/planning	15 min – alert	Keep for self	Prioritize patients
0800				
0830				
0900				
0930				
1000				
1030				
1100				
1130				
1200				
1230				
1300				
1330				
1400				
1430				
1500				
1530				

TABLE 4-2

STRATEGIES FOR AVOIDING TIME-WASTERS

Distraction	Strategies
Casual visitors	Make your environment less inviting. Remain standing. Remove your visitor chair. Keep a pen in your hand.
Unplanned phone calls	Use an answering machine or voice mail. Set a time to return calls.
Unwanted/low priority jobs	Say "No" to jobs that have little value or in which you have little interest. Leave low-priority tasks undone. If an unwanted job must be done, pay or ask for assistance.
Requests for assistance	Encourage others to be more independent. Give them encouragement, but send them back to complete the job. Decisions to help should be conscious decisions, not drop-in distractions.
Clutter	Clear your work area of clutter, and keep it clean. Organize your work area, and take a few minutes at the end of your shift to prepare your area for the next shift.
Interruptions	Open your mail over the garbage can. Respond, delegate, or throw it out. Organize your papers. Keep your notebooks, calendar, and phone lists in one three-ring binder so you have your essentials together.
Procrastination	Break a task down into manageable segments, and return to it again and again until it is complete.
Perfectionism	Become a pursuer of excellence, not a perfectionist, as you pursue your goals (Table 4-3).

TABLE 4-3
BEHAVIORS OF PERFECTIONISTS AND PURSUERS OF EXCELLENCE

Perfectionists	Pursuers of Excellence
• Hate criticism	• Welcome criticism
• Are devastated by failure	• Learn from failure
• Get depressed and give up	• Experience disappointment but keep going
• Reach for impossible goals	
• Value themselves for what they do	• Enjoy meeting high standards within reach
• Have to win to maintain high self-esteem	• Value themselves for who they are
• Can only live with being number one	• Do not have to win to maintain high self-esteem
• Remember mistakes and dwell on them	• Are pleased with knowing they did their best
	• Correct mistakes, then learn from them

Courtesy *Critical thinking in practical/vocational nursing* by L. White (2001). Clifton Park, NY: Delmar Cengage Learning.

EVIDENCE FROM THE LITERATURE

Citation: Standing, T. S., & Anthony, M. K. (2008). Delegation: What it means to acute care nurses. *Applied Nursing Research, 21*(1), 8–14.

Discussion: As health care costs rise, nurses are increasingly delegating tasks to nursing assistive personnel (NAP). The purpose of this phenomenologic study was to describe delegation from the perspective of the acute care nurse. Interviews with staff nurses were completed, and a working definition of delegation was developed using Donabedian's model of structure, process, and outcome to organize the findings. The process of delegation centered on communication and on nurse-NAP relationships and was shaped by the structures on the unit. The outcomes of delegation included nursing and patient outcomes. The authors identified the need for enhanced content on communication and interpersonal relations in nursing education.

Implications for Practice: As nurses seek to incorporate delegation into their practice, they must be given time to develop the skill and education needed to exercise this important skill well. Time must be provided in nursing education programs and in nursing orientation programs for this knowledge and skill development.

EFFECTIVE USE OF AVAILABLE TIME

To plan effective use of available time, nurses must understand the big picture and decide on priority patient outcomes. No nurse works alone. Nurses should know what resources are available, what is expected of their co-workers, what is happening on the other shifts, and what is happening in the organization and the community. If the previous shift was stressed by a crisis on the unit or in the community, a shift may not get started as smoothly (Hansten & Jackson, 2009). If other hospital units outside of a nursing unit are overwhelmed, staff might be moved from one unit to assist on the overwhelmed unit elsewhere in the hospital. When nurses take the big picture into consideration, they are less likely to be frustrated when asked to assist others both on their unit and in the hospital.

SETTING PRIORITY PATIENT OUTCOMES

Nurses set priorities to achieve safe patient outcomes. Priority setting is one of the most critical skills a nurse must develop. Nurses determine priorities by applying the nursing process, assessing the patient, and making a nursing diagnosis. The nurse then plans, implements, and evaluates patient care. This is an ongoing process, calling for constant reassessment and re-prioritization of patient care needs.

Do First Things First. If someone has called in sick and no replacement is available, it might be unreasonable for a nurse to plan to reinforce teaching or discuss the home environment with a patient scheduled to leave the next day. However, there would be no question that interventions that prevent life-threatening emergencies or save a life when a life-threatening event occurs are a priority. They must be done no matter how short the staffing. Nurses must protect their patients and maintain both patient and staff safety, as well as perform the activities essential to the nursing and medical care plans (Hansten & Jackson, 2009).

First Priority: Problems with ABCs. Life-threatening conditions include patients at risk to themselves or others and patients whose vital signs and level of consciousness indicate potential for respiratory or circulatory collapse (Hansten & Jackson, 2009). A patient whose condition is life threatening is the highest priority and requires monitoring until transfer or stabilization. Life-threatening conditions can occur at any time during the shift and may or may not be anticipated.

A quick guide to assessing life-threatening emergencies is as simple as ABC. A stands for Airway. Is the airway open and patent or in danger of closing? This is the highest priority of care. B stands for Breathing. Is there respiratory distress? C stands for Circulation. Is there any circulatory compromise? This is a way of prioritizing actions. Although there is clearly an order of importance, ABC is often assessed simultaneously while observing the patient's general appearance and level of consciousness (Figure 4-3, Table 4-4, and Table 4-5). Patients with

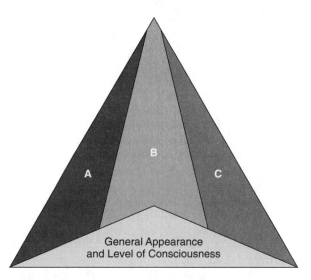

Figure 4-3 Quick assessment tool. (Delmar Cengage Learning.)

TABLE 4-4	
TRIAGE—TOP PRIORITY PATIENTS WITH POTENTIAL THREATS TO THEIR ABCs (EXCERPT)	
Respiratory Patients	• Airway compromise • Choking • Asthma • Chest trauma
Cardiovascular Patients	• Cardiac arrest • Shock • Hemorrhage

(continues)

Table 4-4 *(continued)*

Neurological Patients	• Major head injury • Unconscious • Unresponsive • Seizures
Other Patients	• Major trauma • Traumatic amputation • Major burn, especially if airway involvement • Abdominal trauma • Vaginal bleeding • Anaphylaxis • Diabetic with altered consciousness/ hypoglycemia • Septic shock • Child or elder abuse

Compiled with information from the *Canadian pediatric triage and acuity scale: Implementation guidelines for emergency departments.* Retrieved October 6, 2008, from www.caep.ca

life-threatening conditions usually have an IV access line and receive continuous monitoring of their cardiac rhythm, blood pressure, pulse, respiration, and oxygen saturation level. Their temperature and urinary output are monitored closely as well.

Second Priority: Activities Essential to Safety. Activities that are essential to safety are very important and include those responsibilities that ensure the availability of life-saving monitoring, medications, and equipment, and that protect patients from infections and falls. They include asking for assistance or providing assistance during two-people transfers, or turning and movement of heavy patients (Hansten & Jackson, 2009). They also include monitoring the patient for the prevention of nurse-sensitive outcomes.

Third Priority: Comfort, Healing, and Teaching. Activities that include comfort, healing, and teaching are the activities that, if omitted, will hinder the patient's recovery. These essential activities include nutrition, ambulation, positioning, teaching, and medication administration (Figure 4-4).

Covey, Merrill, and Merrill (2002) developed another way of setting priorities. Activities are classified as urgent or not urgent, as important

TABLE 4-5
IDENTIFYING PRIORITY PATIENTS

- First Priority—ABCs—Remember Maslow's (1970) Hierarchy of Human Needs. Assess physiological needs first. First, examine any high-priority unstable patients who have any threats to their Airway, Breathing, and Circulation (ABCs). These patients require nursing assessment, judgment, and evaluation continuously until transfer or stabilization. Life-threatening conditions can occur at any time during the shift and may or may not be anticipated. Notice your patient's level of consciousness and general appearance. Remember that all equipment and observations used to support and monitor the status of patient's ABCs are also a high monitoring priority, such as monitoring patient suicide threats, vital signs, level of consciousness, neurological status, skin color, temperature, pain, IV access, cardiac rhythm, oxygen, pulse oximetry, suction, urine output, and so on.
- Second Priority—Safety—Assess Maslow's second level of Human Needs, safety and security. Are there any urgent threats to patient safety and security, such as the need for fall prevention, infection control, and so on? See these patients next.
- Third Priority—Comfort, Healing, Teaching—Prioritize the patient's other needs. Patients' nonurgent needs may also include love and belonging, self-esteem, and self-actualization. What do the nursing and medical plan of care include, i.e., comfort, ambulation, healing, teaching, positioning, and so on? Stable patients who need standard, unchanging procedures with predictable outcomes are seen last. Monitoring ABCs and patient safety is always top priorty!

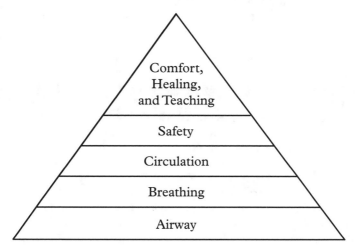

Figure 4-4 Prioritization triangle. (Delmar Cengage Learning.)

or not important. If an activity is neither important nor urgent, then it becomes the lowest priority (Figure 4-5).

Some activities that are often thought of as important may not be. Sometimes laboratory data, vital signs, and intake and output are ordered to be monitored more frequently than the status of the patient indicates. Frequent monitoring of these parameters may make no significant difference in patient outcomes. When nurses begin their shifts, they should question the activities that make no difference in outcomes (Hansten & Jackson, 2009). If a health care provider orders these activities, a nurse should work to get the order changed. Nurses should give priority to the activities that they know are going to make a difference in patient outcomes.

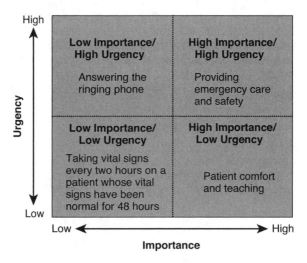

Figure 4-5 Determining priorities. (Delmar Cengage Learning.)

REAL WORLD INTERVIEW

As an emergency nurse, your priorities are very important. Priorities must be flexible to change with the environment. When arriving at work, prepare by checking your patients, rooms, and equipment. Review your patients' charts and receive the Patient Report from the nurse who is going off duty. Then prioritize patient care. Priorities change when new patients arrive or a patient's condition changes. Stay ahead of the curve by anticipating what will happen during the patient's stay. For example, if

(continues)

Real World Interview *(continued)*

a patient's problem is nausea with vomiting, I can anticipate starting the IV and collecting lab samples before the patient sees the MD. When the patient sees the MD and orders are written, the patient can then quickly receive his or her medicine for nausea. I take care of the patient's immediate needs and anticipate his or her future needs.

Chris Curtis, RN
Austin, Texas

Priority Traps.   Vaccaro (2001) states that prioritizing has several traps that nurses should avoid. See Table 4-6.

A frequent prioritizing trap for nurses is the "do whatever hits first" trap. This means that a nurse may want to respond to things that he or she sees first. For example, a nurse at the beginning of the day shift chooses to fill out the preoperative checklist for a patient going to surgery the next day before assessing the rest of the patients.

The second prioritizing trap is the "taking the path of least resistance" trap. In this trap, nurses may make the flawed assumption that it is easier to complete a task themselves rather than delegate it. For example, a nurse who is admitting a patient needs the patient's vital signs, weight, baseline assessment, and patient orders. The first two tasks can be delegated to nursing assistive personnel (NAP) so that the nurse may complete the baseline assessment of the patient and then call the health care provider for orders.

The third prioritizing trap is the "responding to the squeaky wheel" trap, wherein nurses feel compelled to respond to whatever need has been vocalized the loudest. In this case, the nurse may choose to respond to a patient's family member who has come to the nursing station every half-hour

---

TABLE 4-6
PRIORITIZING TRAPS TO AVOID

- Doing whatever hits first
- Taking the path of least resistance
- Responding to the squeaky wheel
- Completing tasks by default
- Relying on misguided inspiration

From *Five priority-setting traps*, by P. J. Vassaro (2001, April). In *Family Practice Management, 8*(4), 60.

with some concern. To appease the family member, the nurse may take time to focus on one of the many expressed concerns and overlook a more pressing need elsewhere.

The fourth prioritizing trap is called "completing tasks by default" trap. This trap occurs when nurses feel obligated to complete tasks that no one else will complete. A common example of this trap is a nurse emptying the garbage instead of asking housekeeping to do it.

The last trap is the "relying on misguided inspiration" trap. The classic example of this trap is when nurses feel "inspired" to document findings in the chart and avoid attending to a higher-priority responsibility. Unfortunately, some tasks will never become inspiring and require discipline, conscientiousness, and hard work to complete them.

KEEP YOUR PATIENTS SAFE 4-2

Nurses set priorities fast when they "First Look" at patients. As you approach your patient, get in the habit of observing the following:

FIRST LOOK
- Eye contact as you approach
- Speech
- Posture
- Level of consciousness

AIRWAY
- Airway sounds or secretions
- Nasal flare

BREATHING
- Rate, symmetry, and depth
- Positioning
- Retractions

CIRCULATION
- Color
- Flushed
- Cyanotic
- Presence of IV or oxygen
- Pain
- Vital signs (TPR and BP)
- Pulse oximetry
- Cardiac monitor

(continues)

Keep Your Patients Safe 4-2 *(continued)*

DRAINAGE

- Urine
- Blood
- Gastric
- Stool
- Sputum

Practice your First Look the next time you approach a patient. Does this improve your assessment skills?

REAL WORLD INTERVIEW

As a triage nurse, I see patients come into the emergency room (ER) ambulatory, by wheelchair, or on a stretcher with Emergency Medical Services (EMS). I see emergent and non-emergent patients and must set priorities. Recognizing and caring for acutely ill or injured patients is our number one priority. These include patients with asthma, chest pain, altered mental status, uncontrolled bleeding, or significant changes in vital signs. These patients need to be taken back to the treatment area first. I also have to monitor the non-emergent patients and let them know they are important and will be cared for in a timely manner. Triage can be very stressful at times, and keeping patients informed is very important.

Karen Woodard, RN
Austin, Texas

PATIENT HANDOFF REPORT, SHIFT ACTION PLAN, AND MAKING ASSIGNMENTS

When the nurse comes on duty, the patient handoff report is given to the oncoming shift by the outgoing shift. At best, a complete report can lead to a smooth and effective start to the shift. At worst, an incomplete report can leave the oncoming shift with inadequate or old data with which to start the patient care plan. There are two ways to deliver patient handoff report—through a face-to-face meeting, or walking rounds. See Table 4-7.

Whether the report is conducted face to face or through walking rounds, priority patient information must be transmitted to allow for the effective and efficient implementation of care. If the outgoing nurse fails to cover all pertinent points, the oncoming shift must ask for the relevant information. See Table 4-8.

TABLE 4-7
PATIENT HANDOFF REPORTS: ADVANTAGES AND DISADVANTAGES

Face-to-Face Reports

Advantages	Disadvantages
• Nurse giving report has actual audience and can include all pertinent information.	• It is time-consuming. It is easy to get side-tracked and gossip or discuss non-patient-related business.
• Nurses get clarification and can ask questions.	• Both oncoming and departing nurses are in report. Patients are not included in planning.

Walking-Rounds Reports

Advantages	Disadvantages
• Provides the prior shift and on-coming shift staff the opportunity to observe the patient while receiving report. Staff can address any assessment or treatment questions.	• It is time-consuming.
• Departing nurse can show assessment and/or treatment data directly to oncoming nurse.	• There is a lack of privacy in discussing patient information.
• The patient is included in the planning and evaluation of care. The information is accurate and timely.	
• Accountability of outgoing care provider is promoted.	
• Patient views the continuity of care as oncoming shift makes initial nursing rounds with prior shift.	

Courtesy *Time Management* by P. Maloney. In *Nursing leadership & management* (2nd ed.) (pp. 281–298), by P. L. Kelly (Ed.) (2008), Clifton Park, NY: Delmar Cengage Learning.

TABLE 4-8
TOOL FOR PATIENT HANDOFF REPORT

		Notes
Demographics	• Room number • Patient name • Sex • Age • Health care provider	
Diagnoses	• Primary • Secondary • Nursing and medical • Surgery/admit date • Pertinent history	
Patient status	• Do Not Attempt to Resuscitate (DNAR) status • Current vital signs • Problem with ABCs, level of consciousness, or safety • Allergies • Oxygen saturation • Pain score • Systems review, as appropriate • Ambulation • Fall risk • Suicide risk • Presence/absence of signs and symptoms of potential complications • New orders/changes in treatment plan	
Diet/IV fluids/ tubes/ oxygen/ laboratory tests and treatments	• Diet • Fluid restriction • Date, IV fluid, rate, site • Tube feedings—Type of tube, contents, rate, and toleration • Oxygen rate, route, other tubes (e.g., chest tube, NG tube, foley, etc.), and drainage	

(continues)

Table 4-8 *(continued)*

	• Abnormal lab and test values • Labs and tests to be done during next shift • Treatments done on your shift, including dressing changes (times, wound description) and procedures • Identify treatments to be done during next shift	
Expected shift outcomes	• Priority outcomes • Patient learning outcomes	
Plans for discharge	• Expected date of discharge • Referrals needed • Progress toward self-care and readiness for discharge	
Care support	• Availability of family or friends to assist in ADL/IADL (activities of daily living/instrumental activities of daily living)	
Priority interventions	• Interventions that must be done this shift	

Nurses strive to expedite reports by focusing on major points of the patient's care and eliminating extraneous information and gossip.

After receiving the patient handoff report, the nurse will consider the shift action plan (Table 4-9). This shift action plan considers the big picture, desired outcomes, shift priorities, interventions, and evaluates patient care for the shift.

MAKING ASSIGNMENTS

After receiving the handoff report and considering the shift action plan, the nurse can complete an assignment sheet: a written or computerized plan that makes assignments to team members and identifies the priorities for the shift. Assignments should include specific reporting guidelines, times for interventions, and deadlines for accomplishing the tasks. Assignments should consider various factors. See Table 4-10. Note the assignment sheet excerpt in Table 4-11.

TABLE 4-9
SHIFT ACTION PLAN

Concern	Consideration
Plan:	
What is the big picture?	How many patients? Any staffing issues? Any environmental concerns?
What are the desired outcomes?	If everything goes well and as expected, what does the nurse hope to accomplish?
	If unexpected setbacks occur, what can the nurse, staff, and patients really accomplish?
What are the priorities?	Who is at greatest risk for potential life-threatening complications? Has all emergency equipment been checked? Are patients who are at a high risk for falls or suicide identified and are measures being taken? Who are the patients suffering from significant symptoms—airway, breathing, circulation?
Intervention:	
What are the "tasks" to be accomplished?	Monitoring? Medication administration? Treatments? Teaching? Counseling? Physical and functional care? Unit support, e.g., stocking, maintenance?
Who is available to do the work, and what skills and attributes do the personnel have?	RN? LPN/LVN? NAP?
What can the RN do? What about the LPN/LVN? What can the NAP do?	RN teaches, counsels, and supervises all nursing care. LPN/LVN can do medication administration and treatments. NAP can complete physical care such as bathing, performing oral care, and obtaining vital signs. Assign and delegate accordingly.
When should the actions be completed by? What are the guidelines for completion?	Give a set time for completion of all tasks.
When are staff breaks/lunch scheduled?	What priority information must be shared with staff, and who is covering patients during breaks/lunch?

(continues)

Table 4-9 *(continued)*

Evaluate:

| Are the shift outcomes achieved? | How will you check throughout the shift and at the end of the shift? Is your team in need of assistance? Has anything unexpected happened to change your plan? Has patient status changed? At the end of the shift, did you accomplish outcomes? |

TABLE 4-10
FACTORS CONSIDERED IN MAKING ASSIGNMENTS

- Priority of patient needs
- Geography of nursing unit
- Complexity of patient needs
- Other responsibilities of staff
- Attitude and dependability of staff
- Need for continuity of care by same staff
- Need for fair work distribution among staff
- Need of patient for isolation and/or protection
- Skill, education, and competency of staff, i.e., RN, LPN/LVN, NAP
- Need to protect patient and staff from injury
- Patient care standards
- Environmental concerns
- Insurance education programs
- Lunch/break times
- Unit routines
- Accreditation regulations
- Agency organizational system
- State laws

MAKING PATIENT CARE ROUNDS

If the patient handoff report does not include walking rounds, the oncoming nurse needs to make initial rounds on the patients at risk for life-threatening conditions or complications first. As the nurse makes rounds, he or she performs rapid assessments. These assessments may vary from the information given in the patient handoff report, so the information gathered on rounds may change the shift plan. For example, a patient with asthma who has been calm and without respiratory distress on the previous shift may have experienced a visitor who wore perfume

CASE STUDY 4-1

Teamwork on a patient care unit—Day shift routine

Throughout the day shift, nursing and unit staff communicate and work together to deliver quality patient care.

7:00 a.m.	Day shift takes patient handoff report from night shift and considers shift action plan
7:15 a.m.	Patient assessment, including vitals, lab work, IVs; charge nurse reviews patient care assignments with all nurses and unit staff; nursing standards, priorities, and goals identified
7:30 a.m.	Breakfast served
7:45 a.m.	A.M. care begins following nursing care standards
8:00 a.m.	Medications administered, health care providers make rounds, patients sent for diagnostic tests, documentation begun, regular patient observations, nursing care standards implemented, e.g., hourly patient rounds, turn Q2H, walk TID, dressing change daily
11:30 a.m.	Vital sign assessment
12:00 p.m.	Lunch served, medications given
2:00 p.m.	Intake and output reports completed; documentation completed
3:00 p.m.	Patient handoff report from day shift to evening shift

How does teamwork get patient care completed? Make out a day shift routine for your clinical unit.

and relayed bad news. As the oncoming nurse makes initial rounds and uses the quick ABC assessment, he or she may quickly determine that the patient has suddenly developed respiratory distress. The patient may have been initially prioritized as requiring only supportive activities directed at healing, but now he or she is experiencing a life-threatening reaction and requires appropriate nursing interventions as well as continuous monitoring.

While assessing all patients, the nurse also checks all the patient IV lines to make sure that the correct fluids are infusing and the infusion sites are without a complication. The nurse checks all the patient drains, tubes, and continuous treatments. The nurse also listens to all patient concerns and desires. It is important to remember that plans are just that, plans, and have to be flexible based on ever-changing patient care needs. Times for treatments and medications may have to be changed. Often nurses believe that the times for administering medication are inflexible, yet health care providers usually write medication orders as daily, twice a day, three times a day, or four times a day. These kinds of orders give nurses flexibility in administration times. Although unit policy dictates when these medicines are given, unit policy is under nursing control.

TABLE 4-11

Assignment Sheet Excerpt   Unit 2 South

Date October 2, 2010

Shift _____ Days _____

Charge nurse _____ Mary _____

RNs Break/Lunch
Steve   0900 and 1100
Lateisha   0930 and 1130
Colleen   1000 and 1200

LPN/LVNs Break/Lunch

NAP Break/Lunch
Juan   0900 and 1100
Pat   0930 and 1130

Notify RN immediately if:

T	<97 or >100
P	<60 or >110
R	<12 or >24
SBP	<90 or >160
DBP	<60 or >100
BS	<70 or >200

Pulse oximetry <95%

Urine output <30 cc/hour

Notify RN one hour prior to end of shift:
I&O
Patient goal achievement

Narcotic Count _____ Steve _____
Glucometer Check _____ Colleen _____
Pass Water _____ Juan _____
Stock Linen _____ Pat _____
Other _____ Colleen to attend in-service at 1300

Room	Patient	Staff	A.M./P.M. Care	Weight I&O	IV	Activity	Accu-check	Tests	NPO	Comments
501, Mr. M. M.	27-year-old with newly diagnosed AIDS, left lower lobe pneumonia	Steve, RN, and Juan, NAP	Complete Care	0715 1400	NS @125 cc/hr.	Bedrest		Lab		Vitals Q4H

(continues)

Table 4-11 *(continued)*

502, Mr. M. G.	61-year-old with acute congestive heart failure (CHF), and diabetes	Lateisha, RN, and Pat, NAP	Partial Bath	0715 1400	KVO	BRP	1100	Lab	Yes	Vitals Q4H
504, Ms. N. J.	48-year-old with new cholelithiasis	Lateisha, RN, and Pat, NAP	Self		KVO	Up ad lib		Ultra-sound	Yes	
505, Ms. L. G.	89-year-old with new onset CVA with right-side paralysis	Colleen, RN, and Juan, NAP	Complete	0715 1400	NS @ 125 cc/hr.	Bedrest	1100	Lab		Vitals Q4H

EVIDENCE FROM THE LITERATURE

Citation: McInnis, L. A., & Parsons, L. C. (2009, December). Thoughtful nursing practice: Reflections on nurse delegation decision-making. *Nursing Clinics of North America, 44*(4), 461–470.

Discussion: This article discusses delegation challenges and legal and regulatory oversight associated with delegation in the clinical practice setting. The authors address moral and legal attributes of the roles and responsibilities of health care providers regarding delegating health care interventions. The article also explores guiding principles and rules of delegation within professional standards, national practice guidelines, and state nurse practice acts. Nurse experts provide thoughtful reflection on nursing models and the role of delegation, emphasizing the critical role of delegation in extending the role of the health care professional in patient care services.

Implications for Practice: Nurses must stay abreast of potential changes in delegation practices. These changes affect the role of the nurse every day.

Evaluating Outcome Achievement

At the end of the shift, the nurse reexamines the assignment sheet. Did the staff and patients achieve the outcomes? It not, why? Were there staffing problems or patient crises? What was learned from this for future shifts?

CASE STUDY 4-2

Nurses use the nursing process as they assess priorities and delegate patient care.

ASSESS

A. You are the RN caring for the following six patients. Patients from another unit that is being painted have been moved to your unit for two days. Use the ABCs to prioritize these patients' needs based on the information given.

Name	Age	Patient Description	Priority Ranking and Rationale
Max Muench	27	Newly diagnosed acquired immune deficiency syndrome (AIDS), has left lower lobe pneumonia	4-Assess respirations and vital signs (VS)

(continues)

Case Study 4-2 *(continued)*

Michael Gray	61	Acute congestive heart failure (CHF) and diabetes, patient ran out of medications a week ago	3-Assess VS and meds
Nirmala Joseph	48	New cholelithiasis, confirmed by ultrasound	6-Assess pain
David Welch	41	New onset unstable angina	1-Assess chest pain and VS
Terry Summer	70	Three days post-hypertensive crisis. BP now 180/102	5-Assess VS and symptoms, e.g., headache
Leona Glusak	89	New-onset CVA with right-side paralysis	2-Assess airway and VS

B. You are working with an LPN/LVN and a NAP. Which of these patient's care could you delegate? (Note that the NAP can stock the unit, give baths, check vitals, and monitor intake and output for all the patients. The LPN/LVN can administer many medications, change dressings, insert foley catheters, etc.). Note that your assessment of staff competence is important as you delegate care. Consider each staff member's education, competence, strengths, and weaknesses as you delegate patient care to assure patient safety. Fill out the assignment sheet in Table 4-12.

C. Is there anything occurring on your unit or on other hospital units that affects your assignments, e.g., have any staff been unable to come to work due to a snow storm? Consider the shift action plan in Table 4-9 as you complete the assignment form in Table 4-12 for all six patients.

PLAN

A. What nursing standards and routines should you apply to these patients? For example:

All patients	Hourly rounds, Q4H vital signs, hygiene, fresh water, new orders, monitoring, safe medication administration, IV monitoring, intake and output, etc.
Bedfast patients	Turn, cough, and deep breathe patients Q2H, intake and output, etc.
Surgical patients	Turn, cough, and deep breathe patients Q2H, routine dressing changes, etc.

B. What health care provider patient orders need to be implemented, e.g., medications, diagnostic tests?

(continues)

TABLE 4-12

ASSIGNMENT SHEET

Unit _____

Date _____
Shift _____
Charge nurse _____
Breaks/Lunch _____
RN _____

LPN/LVN _____

NAP _____

Notify RN immediately if:
T   <97 or >100
P   <60 or >110
R   <12 or >24
SBP <90 or >160
DBP <60 or >100
BS <70 or >200
Pulse oximetry <95%
Urine output < 30 cc/hours or
            240 cc/8 hours

Notify RN one hour prior to
end of shift:
I&O
Patient goal achievement

Narcotic Count _____
Glucometer Calibration _____
Pass Water _____
Stock Linen _____
Code Cart _____
Medication Refrigerator Temperature Check _____
Other _____

Room	Patient	Staff	A.M./P.M. Care	Weight I&O	IV	Activity	Glucom-eter	Tests	NPO	Comments

(continues)

Table 4-12 (continued)

Case Study 4-2 *(continued)*

IMPLEMENT AND EVALUATE
Complete your assignment sheet in Table 4-12. Implement your plan. Monitor patients and environment. Evaluate and change plans as needed. Evaluate if all standards are being met, all orders completed, and all patient and staff outcomes achieved, i.e., patient clinical outcomes, patient and staff satisfaction outcomes, financial outcomes, knowledge outcomes, etc.

KEEP YOUR PATIENTS SAFE 4-3

Four of Marge's patients were discharged today by 10 a.m. The nursing supervisor asked Marge to help out in the ER. Marge agreed and was assigned to help the triage nurse. Identify the order in which patients would be triaged in the ER.
Group I
- A two-year-old boy with chest retractions
- A one-year-old girl choking on a grape
- A five-year-old boy with a knee laceration

You are correct if you see the one-year-old girl choking on a grape first. Remember your ABCs. Patients with airway problems are always seen first. Ideally there is more than one nurse to care for these patients. How about Group II? Which patient should Marge see first?
Group II
- A 60-year-old female who is nonresponsive and drooling
- A 30-year-old male trauma patient who has absent breath sounds in the right side of his chest
- A 15-year-old female who cut her wrist in an attempted suicide

REVIEW QUESTIONS

1. What task should the 3 p.m. to 11 p.m. nurse delegate to the NAP to be completed first?
   A. Restocking the linen closet
   B. Repositioning a patient who is due to be turned
   C. Rechecking vital signs that were elevated at noon
   D. Transporting a patient who is to be discharged to the front door of the hospital

2. The nurse is starting the shift at 11 p.m. What should be delegated to the NAP initially?
   A. Assessing the pedal pulses of a patient who arrived on the floor at 5 p.m., new post-op femoral popliteal graft placement
   B. Passing fresh water to all of the patients
   C. Taking vital signs on assigned patients prior to midnight
   D. Turning off the IV pump alarm that is beeping

3. The nurse has just finished change of shift handoff report. Which patient should the nurse assess first?
   A. A postoperative cholecystectomy patient who is loudly complaining of pain, but received an IV injection of morphine five minutes ago
   B. A postoperative appendectomy patient who will be discharged in the next few hours
   C. A patient with asthma who had difficulty breathing during the prior shift
   D. An elderly patient with diabetes who is on the bedpan

4. The staff RN's assignment on the 7 a.m. to 3 p.m. shift includes a newly admitted patient with pneumonia, a new post-op surgical patient requesting pain medication, and a patient diagnosed with nephrolithiasis who is complaining of nausea. What should the nurse do first after change of shift handoff report?
   A. Assess the newly admitted pneumonia patient.
   B. Give morphine to the new postoperative patient.
   C. Set up the 9 a.m. medications.
   D. Administer Zofran (ondansetron hydrochloride) to the patient complaining of nausea.

5. The nurse has been assigned to a medical-surgical unit on a snowy day. Three of the staff can't make it in to work, and no other staff is available. How should the nurse proceed?
   A. Prioritize care so that all patients get reasonably safe care.
   B. Provide nursing care only to those patients to whom the nurse is regularly assigned.
   C. Have the patient's family and ambulatory patients take care of the other patients.
   D. Refuse the nursing assignment, as the increased number of patients makes it unsafe.

6. The nurse has just completed listening to change of shift handoff report. Which patient will the nurse assess first?
   A. The patient who has a leaking colostomy bag
   B. The patient who is going for a bronchoscopy in two hours
   C. The patient who is in a sickle-cell crisis and has an infiltrated IV
   D. The patient who has been receiving a blood transfusion for the last two hours

7. A new graduate RN who has just received her assignment asks the charge nurse, "Of the list of patients assigned to me, who do you think I should assess first?" What is the best response the charge nurse could make?
   A. "Check the policy and procedure manual for who to assess first."
   B. "Assess the patients in order of their room number to stay organized."
   C. "I would assess the patient who is having respiratory distress first."
   D. "See the patient who takes the most time last."

8. Of the following new patients, who should be assessed first by the nurse?
   A. A patient with a diagnosis of alcohol abuse with impending delirium tremens (DTs)
   B. A patient with a newly casted fractured fibula complaining of pain
   C. A patient admitted two hours ago who is scheduled for a nephrectomy in the morning
   D. A patient diagnosed with appendicitis who has a temperature of 100.2°F orally

9. Which patient should the nurse see first?
   A. The patient who is being discharged in a few hours
   B. The patient who requires daily dressing changes
   C. The patient who is receiving continuous IV Heparin per pump
   D. The patient who is scheduled for an intravenous Pyelogram this shift

10. Which patient task should you delegate to the NAP?
    A. Completing a daily dressing change
    B. Ambulating patients every four hours
    C. Inserting a rectal suppository
    D. Teaching about diabetic diet and insulin requirements

11. The nurse is making out the assignment sheet. Which patient's task is least appropriate to delegate to the NAP?
    A. Assessing patient breathing
    B. Taking blood pressures
    C. Ambulating patients
    D. Transporting patients

12. The NAP asks the nurse if it would be okay to watch the nurse and learn how to do a sterile dressing change on an abdominal wound. What is the best response for the nurse?
    A. "Yes, it is good for you to learn how to do as much as you can."
    B. "Okay, but sterile dressings are only performed by licensed personnel."
    C. "I don't want you to watch, as it makes me nervous."
    D. "Why do you want to watch me?"

13. What task may the nurse delegate to NAP?
    A. Transport a patient on a cardiac monitor to X-ray.
    B. Give tracheotomy care.
    C. Bathe stable patients.
    D. Remove sutures.

14. You received report on the following patients. Who would you make patient care rounds on first?
    A. Patient who is severely allergic to peanuts who just ate potato chips fried in peanut oil
    B. Patient who is now comfortable but has had several episodes of breakthrough pain since the previous day
    C. Patient who is concerned that he had no bowel movement for two days
    D. Patient who is scheduled for pneumonectomy today.

15. The NAP reports to the nurse that a patient with a new laryngectomy is complaining of shortness of breath. What task could be delegated to the NAP by the nurse in this situation?
    A. Listen to the patient's lungs.
    B. Put the patient in Fowler's position.
    C. Suction the patient's tracheotomy tube.
    D. Change the dressing on the patient's incision.

APPLY YOUR SKILLS

1. Practice making assignments with some of the group of patients on the List of Patient Descriptions on page xii of this book. You are the charge nurse and you have two other RNs, one NAP, and one patient sitter on the 3 p.m. to 11 p.m. shift. Your assignment sheet may look like Table 4-13.

   After the first four hours of the shift had passed, the sitter, Jane, put the call light on in Sylvia Thomas's room. The NAP, Jill, answered the call light. Jane requested to take a 15-minute break. Jill notified Steve of the sitter's request. Nurse Steve asked Jill to see if nurse Mary could relieve the sitter. Nurse Mary was in another room with Max Muench, who was beginning to experience difficulty breathing, and nurse Lateisha was checking a blood pressure on Terry Summer. Steve stated that he would not be able to leave his patient just then, and Mary said she thought she could be there in a few minutes. In the meantime, the ER was on the phone ready to give report on a new patient with chronic obstructive pulmonary disease (COPD). Nurse Steve told the NAP, Jill, to keep an eye on the patient Sylvia Thomas, while the sitter went on break. Fifteen minutes later, the sitter, Jane, returned to patient Sylvia Thomas's room. Jane began to scream and yelled for help. The patient had hung herself with her sheets.

TABLE 4-13
MAKING ASSIGNMENTS

Charge Nurse, Steve	RN, Lateisha	RN, Mary	NAP, Jill	Sitter, Jane
Rooms	*Patients*	*Patients*	*Patients*	*Patients*
2504	Summer	Thomas	All	Thomas
2506	Joseph	Muench		
	Collier	Gray		
	Glusak	Welch		
Charge responsibility, including help with all nursing and medical concerns	Total nursing care, including nursing process, orders, medications, IVs, and so on	Total nursing care, including nursing process, orders, medications, IVs, and so on	Complete 3–11 p.m. unit routines, including P.M. care for all patients, distribute water, answer call lights, and so on. Check all patient vital signs at 4 p.m. and 8 p.m.; relieve sitter for dinner; do not leave patient unattended	Suicide precautions; do not leave patient unattended

Nurse Steve asked the NAP, "Jill, how could this have happened? I told you to keep an eye on the patient." Jill replied, "I kept checking in on her." Nurse Steve yelled, "Checking in on her? You were not to leave her alone!"

Was the NAP delegated a duty that was within her job description? How would you have handled this situation when the sitter asked for a break?

2. You go to work one day, and there are too many staff on the unit. Several patients have been discharged. The nursing supervisor asks you to float to another medical-surgical unit. Note the example of the use of priority setting in caring for two patients on this unit. See Table 4-14.

Now, identify the priority nursing assessments for this next group of patients. See Table 4-15.

TABLE 4-14
PRIORITY ASSESSMENTS, GROUP I

Patient	Priority Nursing Assessments
Ms. S. C. is a 92-year-old who is post-op day one after a total hip replacement following a traumatic fall. She is confused and on multiple medications with a history of hypertension and frequent falls. She is anxious and frightened by the "visiting spirits." Her daughter stays with her at all times.	ABCs, vital signs, safety, hip abduction maintained, good dorsolis pedis and posterior tibiolis pulses, level of consciousness, incision/dressing check, and breath sounds. See this patient first during rounds. Safety is a prime concern with this confused patient as well as watching for any postoperative concerns.
Mr. T. S. is a 70-year-old with hypertensive crisis transferred from ICU two days ago. His BP is 180/102, and his cardiac monitor shows occasional premature ventricular contractions.	ABCs, vital signs, cardiac monitor, safety, diet teaching, and pain. See this patient second during rounds. He has a relatively new condition and is on antihypertensive medications.

TABLE 4-15
PRIORITY ASSESSMENTS, GROUP II

Patient	Priority Nursing Assessments
Mr. M. G., a 61-year-old with acute onset of CHF, now complains of chest pain.	
Mrs. L. G., an 89-year-old transferred two hours ago from ICU with a recent brain attack/CVA; nonresponsive, and has right-sided paralysis; family at bedside.	
Mrs. N. J., a 48-year-old with two-day post-op appendectomy; needs teaching about incisional care.	

3. The charge nurse on an adult patient unit assigned each nurse four patients. Lateisha, RN, has just finished her five-month orientation period on the unit. The charge nurse asked Lateisha how she felt about just finishing orientation. Lateisha stated, "I am comfortable with the procedures, routines, and health care provider interactions. I am still having trouble prioritizing what I should do first." The charge nurse assured her that her lack of experience probably had a lot to do with her difficulty prioritizing. The charge nurse went to her locker and gave Lateisha a handy little prioritizing chart the charge nurse has had since she graduated from nursing school. She told Lateisha that she found this quick little reference chart helped her in situations when she was unsure of priorities. Lateisha was grateful for the chart, and she used it that day.

Lateisha was assigned three patients. Mrs. L. G. is an 89-year-old female, transferred two hours ago from ICU with a CVA. She is nonresponsive and has right-sided paralysis. Her family is at her bedside. Lateisha also has Mr. M. G., a 61-year-old male, admitted yesterday with congestive heart failure (CHF) who is complaining of chest pain. She also has Mrs. N. J., a 48-year-old female, who is two-days post-op appendectomy and needs teaching. Use this priority chart to determine whom Lateisha will see first. See Table 4-16.

TABLE 4-16
PRIORITY CHART

Patient Diagnosis	Maslow's Hierarchy of Needs	Priority	Total
	1-ABCs 2-Safety 3-Comfort, healing, and teaching	1-High Importance/High Urgency 2-High Importance/Low Urgency 3-Low Importance/High Urgency 4-Low Importance/Low Urgency	The patient with the lowest total score is seen first by the nurse.
Mrs. L. G., stable, CVA	2	2	4
Mr. M. G., CHF	1	1	2
Mrs. N. J., post-op appendectomy	3	2	5

Based on the total points, Mr. M. G., the patient with the CHF, needs to be assessed by Lateisha first. Based on the priority chart, who should be assessed next?

4. For the next three days, complete an activity log for both your personal time and your clinical work time. On what activities are you spending the majority of time? When is your energy level the highest? Is your energy level related to food intake? What are your biggest time-wasters? How can you schedule your time more productively?

5. Even the simplest priority setting can make a difference in the plan of care for a group of patients. Mary, the 3 p.m. to 11 p.m. nurse, received patient handoff report on her group of patients with a possible admission from the emergency room (ER). Mary prioritized her plan of care. First, she would assess the five patients; second, administer scheduled/prn medications; and third, start documentation of the care she had given so far. As soon as the cafeteria opened, around 4:30 p.m., she would eat her dinner. It would be an early dinner but if she did not eat then, the chance of her getting to the cafeteria after the patient arrived from the ER would be low. Admitting a patient sometimes takes up to two hours to complete. Mary would get very hungry if she did not get a chance to go to the cafeteria when it was open. Taking care of oneself will benefit the patients as well. How do you prioritize and plan your patient care? Do you take care of meeting your own needs as well as your patients'?

 EXPLORING THE WEB

1. If you would like to find a system for managing your time, the following Web sites offer electronic organizers:
www.casio.com
www.sharp-usa.com
www.palm.com

2. If you prefer a less technological time management system, the following Web sites offer nonelectronic organizers and systems for time management:
www.daytimer.com
www.covey.com
www.franklin.com

3. Find a free online calendar that you can access from anywhere:
http://calendar.yahoo.com

4. Look at all the hints and free tools on time management at the Mind Tools Web site. Can you put any of the ideas to use? www.mindtools.com

5. If you find time management an impossible challenge, you can find professional assistance at the Professional Organizers Web site: www.organizerswebring.com

6. Visit this University of Michigan Web site for time management tips: www.umich.edu. Search for "Stress Manager."

7. Point your browser to www.timethoughts.com. Click on "Setting Priorities."

REFERENCES

Canadian pediatric triage and acuity scale: Implementation guidelines for emergency departments. Retrieved October 6, 2008, from www.caep.ca

Covey, S. R., Merrill, A. R., & Merrill, R. R. (2002). *First things first: To love, to learn, to leave a legacy.* New York, NY: Simon & Schuster.

Doffield, C., Gordner, G., & Cathing-Paul, C. (2008, December). Nursing work and the use of nursing time. *Journal of Clinical Nursing, 17*(24), 3269–3274.

Fitzgerald, M., Pearson, A., Walsh, K., Long, L., & Heinrich, N. (2003). Patterns of nursing: A review of nursing in a large metropolitan hospital. *Journal of Clinical Nursing, 12*(3), 326–332.

Grohar-Murray, M. E., & DiCroce, H. R. (2003). Managing resources. In *Leadership and management in nursing* (3rd ed., pp. 291–315). Stanford, CT: Appleton and Lange.

Hansten, R. I., & Jackson, M. (2009). *Clinical delegation skills: A handbook for professional practice* (4th ed.). Sudbury, MA: Jones and Bartlett Publications.

Maloney, P. L. (2008). Time management. In P. Kelly, (Ed.), *Nursing leadership & management* (2nd ed.). Clifton Park, NY: Delmar Cengage Learning.

Maslow, A. H. (1970). *New knowledge in human values.* Washington, DC: Regnery Publishing, Inc., an Eagle Publishing Company.

McInnis, L. A., & Parsons, L. C. (2009, December). Thoughtful nursing practice: Reflections on nurse delegation decision-making. *Nursing Clinics of North America, 44*(4), 461–470.

Mind Tools. (1999–2006). *How to achieve more with your time.* Retrieved February 27, 2006, from www.mindtools.com/tmintro.html

Pareto Principle—The 80–20 Rule—Complete Information. (2008). Retrieved March 1, 2010, from www.gassner.co.il/pareto

Reed, F. C., & Pettigrew, A. C. (2006). Self management: Stress and time. In P. S. Yoder-Wise (Ed.), *Leading and managing in nursing* (4th ed., pp. 413–430). St. Louis, MO: Mosby.

Scharf, L. (1997). Revising nursing documentation to meet patient outcomes. *Nursing Management, 28*(4), 38–39.

Standing, T. S., & Anthony, M. K. (2008, February). Delegation: What it means to acute care nurses. *Applied Nursing Research, 21*(1), 8–14.

Sullivan, E. J., & Decker, P. J. (2004). *Effective leadership and management in nursing.* Lebanon, IN: Pearson.

Upenieks, V. B. (1998). Work sampling: Assessing nursing efficiency. *Nursing Management, 49*(4), 27–29.

Urden, L., & Roode, J. (1997). Work sampling: A decision-making tool for determining resources and work redesign. *Journal of Nursing Administration, 27*(9), 34–41.

Vaccaro, P. J. (2001, April). Five priority-setting traps. *Family Practice Management, 8*(4), 60.

White, L. (2001). *Critical thinking in practical/vocational nursing.* Clifton Park, NY: Delmar Cengage Learning.

SUGGESTED READINGS

Barker, A. M., Sullivan, D. T., & Emery, M. J. (2006). *Leadership competencies for clinical managers.* Sudbury, MA: Jones and Bartlett Publishers.

Cohen, S. (2005). Reclaim your lost time with better organization. *Nursing Management, 36*(10), 11.

Flaherty, M. (1998). The juggling act: Ten tips for balancing work. *Nurseweek.* Retrieved March 5, 2006, from http://www.nurseweek.com/features/98-5/juggle.html

Hendry, C., & Walker, A. (2004). Priority setting in clinical practice: Literature review. *Journal of Advanced Nursing, 47*(4), 427–436.

Jackson, M., Ignatavicius, D. D., & Case, B. (2006). *Conversations in critical thinking and clinical judgment.* Sudbury, MA: Jones and Bartlett Publishers.

Kirkpatrick, C. (2006). Safety first: JC's patient safety goals for *2006. Nursing Spectrum.* Retrieved March 5, 2010, from http://ce.nurse.com/CE583/Safety-First

Marquis, B. L., & Huston, C. J. (2009). *Leadership roles and management functions in nursing: Theory and application* (6th ed.). Hagerstown, MD: Lippincott Williams & Wilkins.

Patterson, E. S., Roth, E. M., Woods, D. D., Chow, R., & Gomes, J. O. (2004). Handoff strategies in settings with high consequences for failure: Lessons for health care operations. *International Journal for Quality in Health Care, 16*(2), 125–132.

Robinson, J., & Godbey, G. (2005). Time in our hands. *The Futurist, 39*(5), 18–22.

CHAPTER 5

Legal Aspects of Patient Care and Delegation

Patricia Kelly, Robyn Pozza-Dollar, Judith W. Martin,
Kathleen Cain, Chad S. Priest, Maureen T. Marthaler

A nurse who concludes that an attending physician has . . . not prescribed the appropriate course of treatment may not modify the course . . . However, the nurse is not prohibited from . . . consulting . . . other(s) . . . concerning those matters, and when the patient's condition reasonably requires it the nurse has a duty to do those tasks . . .

—*Berdyck v. Shinde*, 1993

OBJECTIVES

Upon completion of this chapter, the reader should be able to:

1. Identify selected torts.

2. Discuss negligence and malpractice.

3. Discuss malpractice cases reported in the Professional Negligence Law Reports.

4. Discuss clinical settings of malpractice cases.

5. Describe a health care organization's liabilities other than nursing actions.

6. Identify resources for safe, legal, and ethical nursing practice.

7. Review nursing risks in delegation of patient care.

8. Discuss a checklist to decrease risk of liability.

9. Describe common monetary awards in malpractice cases.

10. Discuss the nurse–attorney relationship in a lawsuit.

Colleen, RN, is busy with four patients. She receives a new intravenous piggyback (IVPB) medication order from the health care provider and orders it from the pharmacy for Max Muench. When the unit clerk tells Colleen that her patient's IVPB medication has arrived from the pharmacy, Colleen quickly grabs the medication and hangs it. A few minutes later, the patient becomes short of breath. As Colleen checks her patient over, she notes to her horror that she hung another patient's IVPB for this patient.

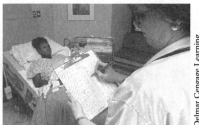

What action should Colleen take immediately?

What should she do next?

What should she do to prevent future errors?

What should the hospital pharmacy and the nursing unit do to prevent future errors?

Is a problem like this the fault of the system, the fault of the nurse, or both?

L aw that governs the relationship between individuals is called **civil law**. Law that specifies the relationship between citizens and the state is called public law. This chapter reviews various laws and common areas of nursing malpractice. It identifies actions a nurse can take to delegate patient care safely and minimize risks to professional practice. It also identifies a nursing checklist to decrease the risk of liability, discusses common monetary awards in malpractice cases, and provides helpful information about the nurse-attorney relationship in a lawsuit.

SOURCES OF LAW

The authority to make, implement, and interpret laws is generally granted in a constitution. A **constitution** is a set of basic laws that specifies the powers of the various segments of the government and how these segments relate to each other.

Generally, it is the role of a legislative body, both on the federal and state levels, to enact laws. Agencies under the authority of the administrative branch of the government draft the rules that implement the law. Finally, the judicial branch interprets the law as it rules in court cases. Table 5-1 gives examples of these relationships.

Also, a judicial decision may set a precedent that is used by other courts and, over time, has the force of law. This type of law is referred to as "common law."

	Legislative Branch	Administrative Branch	Judicial Branch
TABLE 5-1 *THE THREE BRANCHES OF GOVERNMENT*			
Example at federal level	Americans with Disabilities Act (ADA) (1990)	The Equal Employment Opportunity Commission (EEOC) publishes rules specifying what employers must do to help a disabled employee.	In 1999, the U.S. Supreme Court interpreted the law to require that to be protected by this law, the individual must have an impairment that limits a major life activity and that is not corrected by medicine or appliances (e.g., glasses, blood pressure medicine) *Sutton v. United Airlines (1999); Murphy v. United Parcel Service, Inc. (1999)*.
Example at state level	Nurse Practice Act	The state board of nursing develops rules specifying the duties of a registered nurse in that state.	Courts and juries determine whether a nurse's actions comply with the law governing the practice of nursing in a state.

PUBLIC LAW

Public law consists of constitutional law, criminal law, and administrative law and defines a citizen's relationship with government.

CONSTITUTIONAL LAW

Several categories of public law affect the practice of nursing. For example, the nurse accommodates patients' constitutional right to practice their religion every time the nurse calls a patient's clergy as requested, follows a specific religious custom for preparation of meals, or prepares a deceased person's remains for burial.

Controversial constitutional rights that may affect the nurse's practice include the recognized constitutional rights of a woman to have an abortion and an individual's right to die (see *Roe v. Wade* [1973] and *Cruzan v. Director* [1990]). Nurses may not believe in either of these rights personally and may refuse to work in areas in which they would have to assist a patient in exercising these rights. Nurses may not, however, interfere with another person's right to have an abortion or to forgo lifesaving measures.

CRIMINAL LAW

Criminal law focuses on the actions of individuals that can intentionally do harm to others. Often the victims of such abusive actions are the very young or the very old. These two categories of people generally cannot defend themselves against physical or emotional abuse. The nurse, in caring for patients, may notice that a vulnerable patient has unexplained bruises, fractures, or other injuries. Most states have mandatory statutes that require the nurse to report unexplained or suspicious injuries to the appropriate child or elderly protective agency. Generally, the institution in which the nurse is employed will have clear guidelines to follow in such a situation. Failure of the nurse to report the problem as required by law can result in criminal penalties.

Another aspect of criminal law affecting nursing practice is the state and federal requirement that criminal background checks be performed on specified categories of prospective employees who will work with the very young or the elderly in institutions such as schools and nursing homes. Again, this is an attempt to protect the most vulnerable citizens from mistreatment or abuse. Failure to conduct the mandated background checks can result in the institution having to defend itself for any harm done by an employee with a past criminal conviction.

A third area in which criminal law concerns affect nursing practice is the prohibition against substance abuse. Both federal and state law requires health care agencies to keep a strict accounting of the use and distribution of regulated drugs. Nurses routinely are expected to keep narcotic records accurate and current.

Nurses' behavior when off duty can also affect their employment status. Abusing alcohol or drugs on one's own time, if discovered, can result in nurses being terminated from employment and their license to practice nursing restricted or revoked. Frequently, boards of nursing have programs for the nurse with a drug problem, and completion of such a program may be required before the nurse can resume practice. Additionally, health care facilities may require nurse employees to submit to random drug screens to identify those who may be using illegal substances.

ADMINISTRATIVE LAW

Both the federal government and state governments have administrative laws that affect nursing practice. The laws pertaining to Social Security and, more specifically, Medicare, are interpreted in the *Code of Federal*

Regulations, which contains the administrative rules for the federal government. These rules have specific requirements that hospitals, nursing homes, and other health care providers must adhere to if they are to qualify for payment from federal funds. Likewise, state laws are interpreted in administrative rules that specify licensing requirements for health care providers in the state.

Federal. **Administrative law** deals with protection of the rights of citizens. It extends some rights and protections beyond those granted in the federal and state constitutions. An example of this type of law, at the federal level, is the Civil Rights Act of 1964 (1964), which prohibits many forms of discrimination in the workplace. This law may necessitate that the nurse manager make some scheduling accommodations for such things as an employee's religious practices.

Another federal law that affects nursing practice is the Health Insurance Portability and Accountability Act (HIPAA), which was enacted to, among other things, safeguard certain private medical information. Under the law, disclosure of certain protected health information, such as a patient's medical diagnosis or plan of care, can result in criminal penalties. HIPAA is implicated anytime that a patient's private medical information may be shared with another, whether intentional or accidental (Frank-Stromborg, 2004).

Nurses in all practice areas, and of all experience levels, face HIPAA issues each day. For example, large patient information boards were once common features in hospital emergency rooms and inpatient units and were displayed in highly visible areas. On these boards, nurses used to list the names of all the patients on the unit, their nursing and medical health care providers, and perhaps their diagnoses. Today, such a practice

KEEP YOUR PATIENTS SAFE 5-1

You are a new nurse working on the maternal child unit of your local hospital. Your close friend Georgia also got a job on this unit. Georgia has a reputation as a smart, likeable, and hardworking nurse, who also knows how to let loose and have a good time when work is out. However, recently Georgia has been coming to work late and appears "out of it." You spoke with Georgia, who told you that she was having a difficult time at home and had not been as focused at work as she needed to be. She promised that she would try to leave her personal life at home.

For a month after your discussion with Georgia, everything seemed fine. However, in the past two weeks, you have noticed that Georgia has

(continues)

Keep Your Patients Safe 5-1 *(continued)*

had bloodshot eyes, and her speech seems slurred at times. She looks unkempt and unclean, and the narcotic count for Vicodin was off for three separate shifts that she worked. You are concerned that Georgia may be using drugs or alcohol and that it may be impacting her nursing care.

What action do you take? Who can you go to for help in this situation?

might be a violation of HIPAA, as it would disclose the private health information of individual patients. Another example is the chart that many nurses, especially new nurses, use to organize their patient care tasks. Typically these charts identify the patients the nurse is responsible for, their diagnoses, and what medications and treatments they will need. Although these forms are invaluable tools for new nurses learning to organize their clinical practice, they contain sensitive protected health information that, if disclosed, may violate HIPAA. As such, nurses must be on guard to carefully destroy these forms when they are no longer needed (Adams, 2004).

As with most federal laws, the agency responsible for implementing the law has a great deal of power to draft specific rules and regulations. For example, the Occupational Safety & Health Administration (OSHA, n.d.), an administrative agency, works to establish a safe workplace for employees. This includes enacting regulations concerning storage of hazardous substances, protection of employees from infection, and protection of employees from violence in the workplace. Hospitals are subject to numerous OSHA regulations designed to protect the health and safety of nurses and other health care workers. From the minute the new nurse joins the hospital staff, he or she will come into contact with OSHA-mandated products or programs every day. For example, any unvaccinated nurse joining the staff of a hospital will be offered Hepatitis B vaccination pursuant to OSHA regulations. Additionally, nurses working with patients who may have tuberculosis will be issued special OSHA-approved respirators to prevent the nurse from becoming infected. Every day, nurses will utilize OSHA mandated and approved "sharps" containers that hold used needles, and personal protective equipment such as gloves, gowns, and surgical face masks. New nurses should review hospital policies and procedures to ensure they are using these safety devices properly.

State.   An example of a state's administrative law is its nurse practice act. Under nurse practice acts, state boards of nursing are given the authority to define the practice of nursing within certain broad parameters specified by the legislature, mandate the requisite preparation for the practice of nursing, and discipline members of the profession who deviate from the rules governing the practice of nursing. Other professions such as medicine and dentistry have similar practice acts established in state law.

An important issue to nurses is the transferability of their nursing license from one state to another. A license to practice nursing is generally valid only in the state where it is issued. In most cases, a nurse wanting to practice in a state other than where his or her license was issued must apply for a license in that state. For nurses who frequently move from one state to another, this can be a burdensome process. There is an ongoing movement to allow nurses licensed in one state to automatically receive licensure to practice in another state. The Nurse Licensure Compact, a project of the National Council of State Boards of Nursing, is an agreement among states to allow nurses licensed in other states who are parties to the agreement to practice without applying for a new license (Hellquist & Spector, 2004). As of the date of this writing, only 23 states had joined this agreement, meaning that most states still require nurses to apply for a license in the state where they want to practice. You may check the Web to determine if your state is a member of the compact by pointing your browser to www.ncsbn.org. Of course, nurses should always contact the board of nursing in any state where they intend to practice to determine eligibility and licensure requirements.

CIVIL LAW

Civil law governs the relationship between individuals. It encompasses both contract and tort law.

CONTRACT LAW

Contract law regulates certain transactions between individuals and/or legal entities such as businesses. It also governs transactions between businesses. An agreement must contain the following elements to be recognized as a legal contract:

- Agreement between two or more legally competent individuals or parties stating what each must or must not do
- Mutual understanding of the terms and obligations that the contract imposes on each party to the contract
- Payment or consideration given for actions taken or not taken pursuant to the agreement

The terms of the contract may be oral or written; however, a written contract may not be legally modified by an oral agreement. Another way this is often expressed is by the phrase "all of the terms of the contract are contained within the four corners of the document"; that is, if it is not written, it is not part of the agreement or contract. A contract may be express or implied. In an express contract, the terms of the contract are specified, usually in writing. In an implied contract, a relationship between parties is recognized, although the terms of the agreement are not clearly defined, such as the expectations one has for services from the dry cleaner or the grocer.

KEEP YOUR PATIENTS SAFE 5-2

You are assigned to a medical-surgical unit, working the night shift. Your supervisor calls and says that one of the RNs assigned to the critical care unit has called in sick, and you must work that unit instead of your usual assignment. You have never worked in the critical care setting before and have received no orientation to this unit. You are now asked to work there when it is short of staff.

What should you do?

The nurse is usually a party to an employment contract. The employed nurse agrees to do the following:
- Adhere to the policies and procedures of the employing entity.
- Fulfill the agreed-upon duties of the employer.
- Respect the rights and responsibilities of other health care providers in the workplace.

In return, the employer agrees to provide the nurse with the following:
- A specified amount of pay for services rendered.
- Adequate assistance in providing care
- The supplies and equipment needed to fulfill his or her responsibilities
- A safe environment in which to work
- Reasonable treatment and behavior from the other health care providers with whom he or she must interact

This contract may be express or implied, depending on the practices of the employing entity. Sometimes, what is determined to be "reasonable" by the employer is not considered "reasonable" by the nurse. For instance, after 20 years of working as a nurse on the orthopedic unit, a nurse may not view it as reasonable to be pulled to the labor and delivery unit for duty as a nurse there. It would be prudent to express any misgivings to the supervisor and to accept assignments that are in keeping with the experience one has on an orthopedic unit.

TORT LAW

A tort is a negligent or intentional civil wrong not arising out of a contract or statute that injures someone in some way, and for which the injured person may sue the wrongdoer for damages (The 'Lectric Law Library's Lexicon On Tort [2008]). A tort can be any of the following:

1. The denial of a person's legal right,
2. The failure to comply with a public duty, or
3. The failure to perform a private duty that results in harm to another.

A tort can be unintentional, as occurs in malpractice or neglect. It can also be the intentional infliction of harm such as assault and battery. In a tort suit, the nurse can be named as a defendant because of something the nurse did incorrectly or because the nurse failed to do something that was required. In either case, the suit is usually classified as a tort suit. Other tort charges that a nurse may face include false imprisonment, invasion of privacy, and defamation. See Table 5-2.

Nurses must take care to avoid these torts both when they consider nursing action themselves and when they delegate nursing actions to others.

Negligence and Malpractice. If a nurse fails to meet the legal expectations for care, usually defined by the state's nurse practice act, the patient harmed by this failure can initiate an action against the nurse for damages inflicted either by the nurse personally or for damages inflicted by others to whom the nurse has delegated care. **Negligence** is the failure to provide the care a reasonable person would ordinarily provide in a similar situation. The term **malpractice** refers to a professional's wrongful conduct in discharge of his or her professional duties or failure to meet standards of care for the profession, which results in harm to another individual entrusted to the nurse's care.

Simply proving negligence or malpractice is not sufficient to recover damages. Proof of liability or fault requires proof of the following four elements:

1. A duty or obligation created by law, contract, or standard practice that is owed to the complainant by the professional,
2. A breach of this duty, either by omission or commission,
3. Harm, which can be physical, emotional, or financial, to the complainant (patient), or
4. Proof that the breach of duty caused the complained-of harm.

A Louisiana appellate court described the plaintiff patient's specific burden of proof in a negligence or malpractice case against a nurse as:

[T]he three requirements which a plaintiff must satisfy to meet its burden of proving the negligence of a nurse: (1) the nurse must exercise the degree of skill ordinarily employed, under similar circumstances,

TABLE 5-2
SELECTED TORTS

Tort	Definition	Example
Assault	Threat to touch another person in an offensive manner without that person's permission .	Nurse who threatens to give a patient a treatment against his will
Battery	Touching of another person without that person's consent	Nurse who forces a treatment against a patient's will
Invasion of Privacy	All patients have the right to privacy and may bring charges against any person who violates this right	Nurse who shares information about a patient or photographs a patient without consent
False Imprisonment	Restriction of the freedom of an individual	Nurse who restrains a patient who is of sound mind and is not in danger of injuring himself or others
Defamation, Including Libel and Slander	Intentionally false communication or publication, including written (libel) or verbal (slander) remarks that may cause the loss of a person's reputation	Nurse who makes a statement that could either ruin the patient's reputation or cause the patient to lose his job

by the members of the nursing or health care profession in good standing in the same community or locality; (2) the nurse either lacked this degree of knowledge or skill or failed to use reasonable care and diligence, along with her best judgment in the application of that skill; and (3) as a proximate result of this lack of knowledge or skill or the failure to exercise this degree of care, the plaintiff suffered injuries that would not otherwise have occurred (*Odom v. State Dept. of Health and Hospitals*, 1999).

Once a plaintiff presents his or her case, the defendant nurse must show either that if a duty was owed, it was fulfilled, or the nurse must show that the breach of that duty was not the cause of the plaintiff's harm. This must be demonstrated for care delivered by the nurse personally and for care delegated by the nurse to others.

Proving that a duty was owed is not difficult. The plaintiff needs only to show that the nurse was working on the day in question and was responsible either for the plaintiff's care personally or for delegating the plaintiff's care to others. This can usually be accomplished by producing staffing schedules, assignment sheets, job descriptions, policies on delegation, and so on.

To demonstrate a breach of duty, the courts employ a "reasonable man" standard. The test applied for determining this standard is, what would a reasonable and prudent nurse do under the same or similar circumstances? This question is answered by reviewing such documents as the employing organization's policies and procedures, the state nurse practice act, the National Council of State Boards of Nursing (NCSBN) papers on Delegation Decision-Making Tree (NCSBN, 1997), and the Joint Commission's Standards. Testimony from nurses who are accepted as expert witnesses to the standard of nursing practice in the community may also be heard. What is "reasonable and prudent care" can thus be determined from a variety of sources. See Table 5-3.

The defendant nurse's attorney would employ the same methodology to refute the plaintiff's charges. The nurse's attorney would present evidence that the institution's policies and procedures were followed and that the care rendered adhered to accepted nursing standards. To present

---

TABLE 5-3

SOURCES OF EVIDENCE REGARDING A STANDARD OF CARE

- Evidence-based health care research
- Nursing and medical textbooks, articles, and research
- State professional practice acts, i.e., Nurse Practice Act, Physician Practice Act
- Standards of professional association, e.g., American Nurses Association standards
- Equipment manufacturers manuals, e.g., cardiac monitoring equipment manuals
- Written policies and procedures of an organization, e.g., Foley catheter insertion procedures
- Nurse, medical practitioner, or other health care professional expert testimony
- Professional health care accreditation agency criteria, e.g., Joint Commission criteria
- Medication books, e.g., *Physician's Desk Reference, American Society of Health System Pharmacists Drug Information Book,* and so on

the nurse's case, the nurse's attorney would also use expert witnesses to document that the care given or delegated fulfilled the duty owed, was the kind that would be given or delegated by a reasonable nurse in such a circumstance, and that it was not the cause of the plaintiff's harm.

It is not sufficient for a patient plaintiff to show a breach of duty to prevail in a tort suit. He or she must also show that the breach of the duty caused him or her harm. Even if it is proven that a nurse made a medication error or delegated an action incorrectly, if the error was not the cause of the plaintiff's harm, the plaintiff will not win in recovering damages from the nurse. In a recent malpractice case, a patient with sickle-cell anemia died after suffering a cardiopulmonary arrest attributed to an aspiration that was witnessed by a visitor. The visitor immediately called for and obtained help. Although revived, the patient never regained consciousness and was eventually taken off life support. At trial, the plaintiff's attorney was able to prove that the nurse assigned to this patient did not follow the institution's policies in documenting the frequent observations needed by the patient. In reviewing the case on appeal, the appellate court noted:

> [T]he record contains no evidence which suggests what could have been done even if the nurse had been seated at his bedside prior to the arrest. Plaintiff has failed to offer any proof that more immediate assistance would have prevented the catastrophic results of his aspiration. Based on the evidence in this record, we conclude that more frequent monitoring would have made no difference. (*Webb v. Tulane Medical Center Hospital* [1997]).

Thus, even though the plaintiff successfully proved a breach of a duty, the breach was not found to be the cause of the patient's death and the nurse was not found to be guilty of negligence. See Table 5-4 for the types of nursing malpractice cases reported in the *Professional Negligence Law Reporter* from July 2001 through July 2002. Table 5-5 discusses the clinical settings of these nursing malpractice cases. Table 5-6 discusses health care organization liabilities other than nursing actions.

When a nurse is listed as a party in a malpractice lawsuit, the nurse's liability is determined by state laws, such as the nurse practice act, the standards for the practice of nursing, and the institution's policies and procedures. Thus, if the laws mandate that a nurse must have a health care provider's order before doing something, then that order must be present. Problems arise when phone orders are given, and it is later claimed that the nurse misunderstood and acted in error. To prevent this type of malpractice, nurses have adopted the practice of repeating all phone orders back to the health care provider after receiving them and documenting this practice. Another pitfall is illegible writing or the use of inappropriate abbreviations, which are then misinterpreted and the result causes harm to the patient.

TABLE 5-4
*NURSING MALPRACTICE CASES**

Treatment

- Failed to prevent and treat pressure ulcers and malnutrition, resulting in death[5]
- Mishandled shoulder dystocia during delivery, resulting in brachial plexus injury[6]
- Failed to perform intrauterine resuscitation, leading to infant's brain damage[11]
- Failed to properly handle telephone triage calls, resulting in death[12]
- Failed to incorporate patient's emergency room records into patient's hospital chart, resulting in death[12]
- Failed to properly treat pediatric glaucoma, resulting in vision loss[13]
- Burned patient with hair dryer, resulting in third-degree burns[15]
- Failed to accurately count sponges after operation, resulting in retained sponge[16]
- Failed to provide adequate nutrition and implement nursing plan of care, resulting in death[19]
- Injected patient with used needle, leading to emotional distress from possible hepatitis infection[23]
- Failed to properly treat patient's jaundice, resulting in infant's brain damage[24]
- Failed to treat dehydration and pressure ulcers, resulting in death[27]
- Removed internal pacemaker wires improperly, resulting in infection[29]
- Administered suction tube improperly, leading to aspiration and death by suffocation[30]
- Failed to detect arterial blockage after surgery, leading to leg amputation[32]
- Failed to adequately hydrate patient prior to Cesarean delivery, resulting in maternal hypotension and infant's brain damage[33]
- Failed to administer supplemental oxygen, resulting in vision loss and brain damage[44]

Communication

- Failed to notify health care provider of
  a. Patient burns[15]
  b. Bleeding gastric ulcer, resulting in death[9]
  c. Increased heart rate, resulting in death[14]
  d. Fetal distress, resulting in death or brain damage[3, 17, 22]
  e. Newborn jaundice, resulting in brain damage[24]
  f. Pain and numbness after spinal surgery, resulting in cauda equina syndrome[39]
  g. Vision problems, resulting in vision loss[40]

(continues)

Table 5-4 *(continued)*

- Failed to report sexual abuse of patient/resident to police and/or state department of human resources[10, 31]
- Failed to institute chain of command when health care provider refused to come to the hospital promptly[26, 37]

Medication

- Administered insufficient Heparin, leading to death by pulmonary embolism[1]
- Administered doses of Dilantin and insulin to a patient in excess of health care provider's order, leading to patient's disorientation and burns by bedside heater[4]
- Administered excessive dose of IV antibiotics (Nafcillin), leading to chemical burn[18]
- Failed to recognize dosage error in health care provider's order and thereby administered excessive dose of Dilaudid, leading to brain damage[36]

Monitoring/Observing/Supervising

- Failed to monitor premature newborn, leading to death by cardiac arrest[2]
- Failed to monitor patient, leading to third-degree burns[4]
- Failed to timely call a "code blue" in response to patient's respiratory arrest, resulting in death[7]
- Failed to prevent patient falls, leading to death or quadriplegia or quadriparesis[8, 42, 43]
- Failed to seek timely medical intervention, leading to death from bleeding ulcer[9]
- Failed to properly monitor heart rate after surgery, resulting in death[14]
- Misidentified and mixed up newborns in nursery[20]
- Failed to monitor respiratory rate after surgery, resulting in death[21]
- Failed to record vital signs of patient in waiting room, resulting in brain damage[34]
- Failed to restrain demented patient, resulting in death[35]
- Failed to properly insert Foley catheter during delivery, resulting in urinary sphincter trauma and incontinence[38]
- Failed to monitor cornea in facial palsy, leading to corneal scarring and vision loss[40]
- Failed to reattach cardiac monitor after X-rays, resulting in death[41]
- Failed to detect brain swelling, resulting in vision loss and diminished I.Q.[45]

*Reported in *Professional Negligence Law Reporter*, July 2001 through July 2002 (Courtesy Pozza, R. (2003). Unpublished manuscript.)

TABLE 5-5
*CLINICAL SETTINGS OF NURSING MALPRACTICE CASES**

Clinical Setting	No. of Cases
Hospital-Medical-Surgical[7, 15, 16, 18, 21, 25, 29, 32, 36, 39, 40, 43, 45]	13
Maternity-Obstetrics[3, 6, 11, 17, 22, 26, 33, 38, 46, 47]	10
Nursing Home[4, 5, 8, 9, 19, 27, 30, 31, 35]	9
Emergency Room[1, 12, 23, 41, 42]	5
Pediatrics-Nursery[2, 20, 24, 28]	4
Recovery Room[14, 37]	2
Home Health Care[10, 44]	2
Clinic[13]	1
Urgent Care Facility[34]	1
Total	**47**

*Reported in *Professional Negligence Law Reporter*, July 2001 through July 2002 (Courtesy Pozza, R. (2003). Unpublished manuscript.)

TABLE 5-6
*HEALTH CARE FACILITY LIABILITIES OTHER THAN NURSING ACTIONS**

- Failure to provide a safe environment[4, 30, 35]
- Misrepresenting level of care available at nursing home[5]
- Failure to adequately train personnel in fall prevention[8]
- Failure to adequately supervise nursing home staff to ensure residents received proper nutrition, custodial treatment, and medical care[19]
- Failure to instruct and train personnel regarding the handling of jaundice in newborns[24]
- Failure to adequately train staff on emergency procedures[34]
- Failure to inform health care provider of patient burns[15]
- Failure to properly supervise staff[10, 19]
- Failure to provide timely lab services[23]
- Failure to appropriately dispose of used syringes[23]
- Failure to enforce policies to adequately handle emergencies[30]
- Failure to report abuse of nursing home resident[31]
- Allowing unlicensed persons to administer IV medications[34]

*Reported in *Professional Negligence Law Reporter*, July 2001 through July 2002 (Courtesy Pozza, R. (2003). Unpublished manuscript.)

See www.jointcommission.org, click on "Patient Safety" and then, click on the "Do Not Use" list for the JC's list of abbreviations to avoid.

Nurses who have been in practice for a long time have encountered health care providers who write orders that are contrary to accepted practice. In these situations, the nurse must exercise professional judgment and follow the policies and procedures of the institution. Usually these require the nurse to clarify the order with the health care provider and discuss the order as needed with the nursing supervisor and the medical director for the area in which the nurse works in order to clarify it (Martin, Cain, & Priest, 2008).

As mentioned earlier, practicing nurses must also adhere to the standards of practice for the nursing profession in the community. These standards include checking the six "rights" of medication administration (the right patient, medication, dose, time, route, and documentation). If staffing is poor or the nurse receives poor evaluations for taking too long to deliver care, the nurse must identify what standards to follow to preserve professional nursing practice, to protect patients, and to keep the nurse from liability. Seeking help early and maintaining clear communication with other health care providers and the supervisors whom one works with help to limit the nurse's exposure to liability.

Nursing Advocacy.   The American Nurses Association Code of Ethics and many state nurse practice acts require nurses to serve as patient advocates (ANA, 2001b). A patient's illness, combined with the institutional nature of hospitals, often results in him or her becoming a passive recipient of health care instead of an active partner. Nurses are often called upon to help patients communicate their desires and needs to the health care team and to be vigilant in protecting patients' safety and legal rights. For example, occasionally a provider's order may appear suspect or clearly contrary to accepted medical practice. In such situations, the nurse must exercise professional judgment and refuse to carry out the order if it would put the patient in danger. Most organizations have policies and procedures to assist the nurse in carrying out this advocacy function. These procedures often require the nurse to take the issue up the "chain of command," from the nursing manager up through the medical staff if necessary. Nurses are increasingly being held liable for negligence in failing to question potentially improper provider orders.

Nurses also serve as advocates by safeguarding patient legal interests, such as the right to make informed health care decisions. In this role, nurses frequently collaborate with other members of the health care team and provide patient education to ensure that patients understand the risks and benefits of procedures, medication regimens, or laboratory tests. Additionally, nurses may help patients express their desires regarding end-of-life deci-sions to the medical team. Both of these issues are discussed in detail later in this chapter.

It is not uncommon for a nurse to find conflicts between an employ-er's expectations and the nursing standard of care. A nurse working in a medical-surgical ward may be asked to take care of an unsafe number of patients, or a surgical nurse with no experience working in the ER may be asked to "float" to this unit. In these situations, nurses must advocate on behalf of their patients and their profession, and consider whether it is ap-propriate to take on such an assignment. The nurse must maintain patient safety and notify the supervisor and other appropriate representatives from the chain of command, as needed.

Assault and Battery. Assault is a threat to touch another in an offensive manner without that person's permission. Battery is the touching of another person without that person's consent. In the health care arena, issues of this nature usually pertain to whether the individual consented to the treat-ment administered by the health care professional. Most states have laws that require patients to make informed decisions about their treatment.

Informed consent laws protect the patient's right to practice self-determination. The patient has the right to receive sufficient information to make an informed decision about whether to consent to or refuse a pro-cedure. The individual performing the procedure has the responsibility of explaining to the patient the nature of the procedure, benefits, alternatives, and the risks and complications. The signed consent form is used to docu-ment that this was done, and it creates a presumption that the patient had been advised of the risks.

Often the nurse is asked to witness a patient signing a consent form for treatment. When you witness a patient's signature, you are vouching for two things: that the patient signed the paper and that the patient knows he is signing a consent form. For a consent form to be legal, a patient, in most states, must be at least 18-years-old; be mentally competent; must know the procedures, with their risks and benefits, explained in a manner he can understand; be aware of the available alternatives to the proposed treatment; and consent voluntarily. The nurse must also be familiar with which other people are allowed by state law to consent to medical treat-ment for a patient when he or she cannot consent for himself. Frequently, these include the person possessing medical power of attorney; a spouse; adult children; or other relatives, if no one is available in one of the other categories listed.

A nurse may also face a charge of battery for failing to honor an advance directive, such as a medical power of attorney, durable power of attorney, or living will. Federal law requires that a hospital ask the patient, upon admission, whether she has a living will; if she does not, the hospital must ask the patient whether she would like to enact one. A living will is a written advance directive voluntarily signed by the patient that specifies the type of care she desires if and when she is in a terminal state and cannot sign a consent form or convey this information verbally. It can be a general statement such as "no life-sustaining measures" or specific such as "no tube feedings or respirator." Often, the patient's family has difficulty allowing health care personnel to follow the wishes expressed by the patient in a living will, and conflicts arise. These should be communicated to the hospital ethics committee, pastoral care department, risk management, or whichever hospital department is responsible for handling such issues. If the patient verbalizes her wishes regarding end-of-life care to her family, such difficult situations can sometimes be avoided. The patient should be encouraged to do this, if possible.

The nurse should be familiar with the requirements for the implementation of a advertice directives in the state where the nurse practices.

Do Not Attempt to Resuscitate (DNAR) Orders and Following Orders. The attending health care provider may write a Do Not Attempt to Resuscitate (DNAR) order on a patient, which directs the staff not to perform the usual cardiopulmonary resuscitation (CPR) in the event of a sudden cardiopulmonary arrest. The health care provider may write such an order without evidence of Advance Directives on the medical record, and the nurse should be familiar with the organization's policies and state law regarding when and how a health care provider can write such an order in the absence of an advance directive. Often, a DNAR order is considered a medical decision that the doctor can make, preferably in consultation with the family, even without an executed advance directive by the patient.

If the nurse feels that a DNAR order or any order is contrary to the patient's good, the nurse should consult the policies and procedure of the institution. As identified in Chapter 1, these policies include going up the administrative chain of command until the nurse is satisfied with the course of action and has assured patient safety. This may entail notifying all the health care providers, the charge nurse, the nursing supervisor, the nursing director, the medical director, the risk manager, the organization's chief operating officer, state regulators, and/or the accrediting agency, i.e., the joint commission. Often an organization has an ethics committee that may examine such issues and make a determination of the appropriateness of the order.

REAL WORLD INTERVIEW

I took care of a postoperative patient who developed a wound infection when his incision did not heal after a wound dehiscence that was left open to heal on its own. I worked with this patient's health care provider on a regular basis on the unit where I was assigned. The health care provider told me that he was just going to watch the patient for a while, as he thought the wound dehiscence would heal by itself. This did not happen and I lost faith in the health care provider, as the patient was doing poorly. I talked again with the patient's health care provider who continued to say that he was just going to watch the patient. I mentioned to the health care provider that I was concerned about the patient and was going to discuss my concerns with the supervisor, hoping the health care provider would respond to this gentle nudge and take the initiative and do something more for the patient. I had worked with this health care provider for a long time. When he did not take any action, I reported my concerns to my supervisor. The supervisor reported the situation to the Director of Nursing, who discussed the case with the Chief of the Medical Staff. The Chief of the Medical Staff then discussed the case with the original health care provider who agreed to ask another surgeon for a consultation. They did this and took the patient back to surgery. While I was happy for the patient who did well, I felt bad about my relationship with the original health care provider, whom I continued to work with daily. He never spoke to me again. I know I did the right thing. I wish it were easier.

Kelly, RN
Chicago, Illinois

FALSE IMPRISONMENT

A claim of false imprisonment may be based on the inappropriate use of physical or chemical restraints. Federal law mandates that health care organizations employ the least restrictive method of ensuring patient safety. Physical or chemical restraints are to be used only if necessary to protect the patient from harm when all other methods have failed. If the nurse uses restraints on a competent person who is refusing to follow the health care provider's orders, the nurse can be charged with false imprisonment or battery. If restraints are used in an emergency situation, the nurse is to contact the health care provider immediately after application to secure an order for the restraints. Also, the nurse must check the organization's policies regarding the type and frequency of assessments required for a patient in restraints and how often it is necessary to secure a reorder for the restraints. These policies ensure the patient's safety and must be consistent with state law.

False imprisonment occurs when individuals are incorrectly led to believe they cannot leave a place. This often occurs because the nurse misinterprets the rights granted to others by legal documents such as power of attorney and does not allow a patient to leave a facility because the person with the power of attorney (agent) says the patient cannot leave. A power of attorney is a legal document executed by an individual (principal) granting another person (agent) the right to perform certain activities in the principal's name. It can be specific, such as "sell my house," or general, such as "make all decisions for me, including health care decisions." In most states, a power of attorney is voluntarily granted by the individual and does not take away the individual's right to exercise his or her own choices. Thus, if the principal (patient) disagrees with his or her agent's decisions, the patient's wishes are the ones that prevail. If a situation occurs in which an agent, acting on a power of attorney, disagrees with your patient regarding discharge plans, contact your supervisor for further assistance in deciding an action consistent with your patient's wishes and best interests.

The authority to make medical decisions for another may be granted in a general power of attorney document or in a specific document limited to medical decisions only, such as a medical power of attorney. The requirements for a medical power of attorney vary from state to state, as do most legal documents.

CASE STUDY 5-1

You are working the night shift. The health care provider has ordered a dose of a medication that you know is too high to be given to the patient. You are unable to contact the health care provider to check the order. What would you do to ensure safe care for your patient?

Invasion of Privacy. The nurse is required to respect the privacy of all patients. The nurse may be privy to very personal information and must make every effort to keep it confidential. This often necessitates policing conversations with co-workers that have the potential for being overheard by others so that no patient information is accidentally revealed. Sometimes the protection of a patient's privacy conflicts with the state's mandatory reporting laws for the occurrence of specified infectious diseases such as syphilis or human immunodeficiency virus (HIV). The need to protect an individual's privacy may also conflict with the state's mandatory reporting laws on suspected patient abuse, discussed previously. Other information that state or federal law may require to be revealed include a patient's blood alcohol level, incidences of rape, gunshot wounds, and adverse reactions to certain drugs. Failing to strictly follow reporting laws could lead to criminal, civil, or disciplinary action; termination of employment; or all of these. Nurses must consult the institution's policies and confer with its risk management department to ascertain their responsibilities and course of action. The ANA Code of Ethics for Nurses (ANA, 2001a) states that nurses must protect the patient and the public when incompetence or unethical or illegal practice compromises health care and safety. Many states have adopted this concept in their nurse practice acts, thereby creating a legal obligation to report. Nurses who observe unethical behavior in a hospital should report it as directed in the institution's policies and procedures manual or by the laws of the state.

RESOURCES FOR SAFE, LEGAL, AND ETHICAL NURSING PRACTICE

There are many resources that assist nurses in determining what is safe nursing practice. Nurses should be familiar with these in performing their duties. A few key resources are discussed here.

STATE NURSE PRACTICE ACT

The nurse practice act in each state specifies the legal parameters of nursing practice in that state. It answers questions regarding what a nurse can legally do in that state, which may differ from other states. The nurse must know what a nurse is allowed to do in the state where he or she practices. It is not sufficient to say, "I know how to do this, and I was allowed to do it in Nebraska." If a practice is not within the scope of nursing as it is defined in Mississippi, the nurse cannot do it in Mississippi. For access to state boards of nursing, consult the Web site www.ncsbn.org.

POLICIES AND PROCEDURES OF THE INSTITUTION

In most conflicts regarding nursing care, the organization's policies and procedures are examined and are usually admitted as evidence of what the nurse is expected to do. Failure to follow the policies and procedures of the organization in providing care can expose the nurse to personal liability without the protection of the institution. Nurses must know the policies and procedures of their employers and adhere to these in everyday practice.

GOOD SAMARITAN LAWS

Good Samaritan Laws are laws that have been enacted to protect the health care professional from legal liability for actions rendered in an emergency when the professional is providing service without pay. The essential elements of the commonly enacted Good Samaritan Law are:

1. The care is rendered in an emergency situation,
2. The health care worker is rendering care without pay, and
3. The care provided did not recklessly or intentionally cause injury or harm to the injured party.

Note that Good Samaritan Laws are intended to protect the volunteer who stops to render care at the scene of an accident. They would not protect a nurse, Emergency Medical Technician (EMT), or other health care professional rendering care at the scene of an accident as part of their assigned duties and for which they receive pay. These paid emergency personnel would be evaluated according to the standards of their professions in doing their duties (Martin, Cain, & Priest, 2008).

GOOD COMMUNICATION

The nurse must communicate accurately and completely both verbally and in writing. Many lawsuits result from a lack of communication by the nurse or other health care providers. Either the nurse failed to monitor the patient and notify the health care provider of a change in the patient's status, or the nurse failed to document assessments performed or failed to demonstrate competent, caring nursing practice to the patient. It is essential that the nurse communicate thoughtfully with the patient and chart accurately and completely. Patients are less likely to sue if they feel that a nurse has been caring and professional. Often a case involving patient care takes several years to come to trial. By that time, the nurse may have no memory of the incident in question and must rely on the written record created at the time of the incident. This record is frequently in the courtroom, blown up to billboard size for all to see. All errors are apparent and omissions stand out by their absence, especially if the documentation is something that should have been recorded per the organization's policy. The old adage that "if it wasn't documented, it wasn't done" will be repeated to the jury numerous times.

REAL WORLD INTERVIEW

Most nurses are familiar with the phrase, "If it was not documented, it was not done." Insofar as this phrase is used to encourage thorough documentation, it reflects good nursing practice. Timely, accurate, and complete documentation is an excellent way to protect oneself from litigation. However, lawyers who represent plaintiffs in medical malpractice cases

(continues)

Real World Interview *(continued)*

are aware of this "rule" and often attempt to use it unfairly against nurses in health care liability claims.

Imagine the following scenario: A patient is admitted to the hospital, and Nurse A performs an initial assessment of the patient. Nurse A notes in the patient's chart that the patient has good capillary refill. Nurse A proceeds to record the patient's vital signs, including capillary refill, hourly throughout Nurse A's eight-hour shift. The patient's capillary refill remains good, and the nurse makes no further documentation in the chart relating to the patient's capillary refill. After Nurse A's shift, Nurse B takes over the patient's care. One hour into Nurse B's shift, the patient codes and expires. The patient's family sues Nurse A. The plaintiffs' lawyer is cross-examining Nurse A.

Lawyer: "Nurse A, are you familiar with the phrase, 'If it wasn't documented, it wasn't done'?"

Nurse A: "Yes."

Lawyer: "That's a common rule in nursing practice, isn't it?"

Nurse A: "Yes."

Lawyer: "You were taught that in nursing school, weren't you?"

Nurse A: "Yes, I was."

Lawyer: "And after you documented that the patient had good capillary refill upon admission, you did not document anything relating to the patient's capillary refill for the next eight hours, did you?"

Nurse A: "Well, no."

Lawyer: "So if we use your rule, 'If it wasn't documented, it wasn't done,' we can assume you never checked the patient's capillary refill during your shift after the initial assessment, right?"

Nurse A: "No. I checked, but it hadn't changed, so I didn't document anything . . ."

Notice what just happened in the above exchange. Nurse A provided competent nursing care, but the lawyer made it appear as if Nurse A was negligent. A nurse involved in litigation should not blanketly agree with the documentation rule. You simply cannot document everything noted in an assessment of a patient. Moreover, most nurses would agree that patient care takes priority over documentation. This rule ignores that. Bad documentation looks bad. Good documentation protects you. Lapses in documentation do not correlate with bad nursing care, however. Nurses should not lose sight of that when faced with litigation.

Robyn D. Pozza-Dollar, JD
Austin, Texas

EVIDENCE FROM THE LITERATURE

Citation: Croke, E. M. (2003). Nurses, negligence, and malpractice. *American Journal of Nursing, 103*(9), 54–64.

Discussion: This article discusses the actions that prompted charges of negligence that led to malpractice lawsuits against nurses from 1995 to 2001. It identifies several factors that have contributed to the increase in malpractice cases against nurses. According to the National Practitioner Data Bank (NPDB, n.d.), 2,311 nonspecialized nurses made malpractice payments in cases reported to NPDB, 1995–2001. Annual reports of the NPDB are available at www.npdb-hipdb.com. The author states that the majority of payments by nonspecialized nurses in malpractice suits resulted from problems relating to monitoring, treatment, medication, obstetrics, and surgery. Negligence areas discussed include failure to act as a patient advocate; failure to communicate adequate information to the health care provider or patient; inadequate patient assessment, nursing interventions, or nursing care; medication errors; inadequate infection control; failure to document; and unsafe or improper use of equipment. Monetary awards were paid either directly by independent practitioners or by employers according to the doctrine of respondeat superior. The author also discusses strategies for reducing potential liability.

Implications for Practice: Knowledge of the legal implications of nursing practice is necessary to assure that you are taking proper action to reduce your liability.

Documentation. Professional responsibility and accountability are two primary reasons why nurses document. Other reasons to document include communication, education, research, meeting legal and practice standards, and reimbursement. Documentation is the professional responsibility of all health care practitioners. It provides written evidence of the nurse's accountability to the patient, the organization, other health care professionals, and society. Thorough documentation provides:

- Accurate data needed to plan the patient's care in order to ensure continuity of care
- A method of communication among the health care team members responsible for the patient's care
- Written evidence of what was done for the patient, the patient's response, and any revisions made in the plan of care
- Compliance with professional practice standards, e.g., American Nurses Association
- Compliance with accreditation criteria, e.g., Joint Commission (JC), Healthcare Facilities Accreditation Program (HFAP), etc.

- A resource for review, quality improvement, reimbursement, education, and research
- A documented legal record to protect the patient, organization, and nursing and medical practitioners. See Table 5-7.

For protection when charting, the nurse should use the FLAT (Factual, Legible, Accurate, and Timely) charting acronym. See Table 5-8.

TABLE 5-7

NURSING CHECKLIST FOR DOCUMENTATION

Reviewing a Chart

- Can the assessment data that triggered the nursing diagnosis be identified?
- When the defining characteristics of a specific nursing diagnosis are compared to the patient's presenting signs and symptoms, is there supporting evidence?
- Were critical questions asked during the patient interview?
- Did the nurse use the data obtained from both the interview and physical assessment in establishing the diagnosis?
- Can any assumptions that might have misled the nurse's judgment be identified?
- Are the nursing data correlated with the results of the physical examination and findings from diagnostic tests?
- Are the expected outcomes realistic?

From *Fundamentals of Nursing* (4th ed.), by S. C. DeLaune and P. K. Ladner, 2011, Clifton Park, NY: Delmar Cengage Learning.

TABLE 5-8

FLAT CHARTING

F: Charting should be **F**actual—what you see, not what you think happened.

L: Charting should be **L**egible, with no erasures. Corrections should be made with a single line drawn through the error and initialed.

A: Charting should be **A**ccurate and complete. What color was the drainage and how much was present? How many times, and at what times, was the doctor notified of changes?

T: Charting should be **T**imely—completed as soon after the occurrence as possible. Late entries should be avoided or kept to a minimum.

Electronic Health Records.   Several hospitals have adopted electronic health records (EHRs). EHRs eliminate paper record storage and improve access to patient records, in addition to controlling legibility and promoting timely capture of data. An EHR can also be used to gather data about patient care and outcomes, staff activities, and other data for clinical, administrative, and financial decision making.

The U.S. Department of Veterans Affairs (VA) has the largest EHR, known as the Veterans Health Information System and Technology Architecture (VistA). Health care providers can review and update a patient's EHR at any of the over 1,000 VA organizations nationwide. VistA's EHR allows practitioners to place orders, including medication, diet, lab, and X-ray, orders, etc. The U.S. Indian Health Service has an EHR that is similar to VistA. In 2005, the United Kingdom implemented an EHR, designed to provide access to 60,000,000 patients' EHR by 2010. In 2005, the Canadian province of Alberta began an EHR project, which is expected to encompass all of Alberta (Electronic health record, 2008). Implementation of an EHR has been slowed in the U.S. because of concerns over several legal barriers, i.e., paper-era state regulations that may not permit EHRs, antikickback statutes, Stark antireferral rules, concerns about malpractice exposure, HIPAA, antitrust laws, etc. (Shay, 2005).

EVIDENCE FROM THE LITERATURE

Citation: Austin, S. (2006). Ladies and gentlemen of the jury, I present . . . the nursing documentation. *Nursing, 36*(1), 56–64.

Discussion: Poor nursing documentation will undermine your credibility if you are ever involved in a lawsuit. Avoid these red flags in your documentation: Evidence of:
- Lack of treatment
- Delayed, substandard, or inappropriate treatment
- Lack of patient teaching or discharge instructions
- Charting inconsistencies, such as lapses in time
- References to an incident report
- Patient abandonment or patient bias
- Battles between health care providers
- Lack of informed consent
- Late entries that aren't documented as such, or that appear to be self-serving rather than genuine addendums
- Fraudulent or improper alterations of the record

(continues)

Evidence from the Literature *(continued)*

- Destruction of records or missing records
- Failure to accurately assess and monitor the patient's condition
- Failure to notify the health care provider of problems
- Failure to follow orders
- Contributing to medication errors
- Failure to ensure patient safety
- Failure to follow policies and procedures
- Failure to properly delegate and supervise

Implications for Practice: Nurses should avoid these documentation errors. Good documentation habits protect a good nurse.

ETHICAL BEHAVIOR

The nurse's role as a patient advocate and adherent of ethical behavior can help the nurse avoid being named in a lawsuit, as well as help the nurse maintain quality nursing care. Nurses often intervene on behalf of patients in the implementation of health care by notifying a nursing or medical practitioner of a patient problem, scheduling treatment by other departments, referring appropriately, explaining how the system works, assisting with follow-up activities, reinforcing health teaching, coordinating care, preparing for safe discharge, and notifying appropriate individuals of patient needs. The nurse plays a unique role in the delivery of health care in acting as the intermediary between the patient and the health care system. The nurse is often the key person involved in identifying a patient problem and ensuring the patient access to appropriate quality health care. Nurses who advocate for their patients, and who maintain good communication with them and follow ethical principles and rules in an ethical workplace will have little problem with malpractice. See Tables 5-9 and 5-10.

EVIDENCE FROM THE LITERATURE

Citation: Vonfrolio, L. G. (2006, October). Blow the whistle? *RN, 69*(10), 60.

Discussion: When a nurse "blows the whistle" on an unsafe situation, there are often professional consequences. The nurse may be labeled a "troublemaker," isolated from his or her peers, or, worse yet, fired. Currently, fewer than half of the states in this country offer whistleblower

(continues)

Evidence from the Literature *(continued)*

protection. Proceed with caution if you are planning on blowing the whistle. Be sure to:

- Document the incident(s) and keep a copy for yourself. Send a typed complaint to the Director of Nursing (DON) or anyone in another department with a stake in the case.
- Avoid being confrontational when discussing the issue with management. Exhaust all internal remedies before taking matters out of house.
- Keep a personal diary of events after the incident is reported.
- Seek the support of your colleagues. Nurses must band together to protect patients from incompetent, unethical, or unsafe care.
- Consider reporting your concerns about quality of care to the Joint Commission at: www.jointcommission.org. Click on "Report a Complaint" at the bottom of the home page, or send an e-mail to complaint@jointcommission.org. If you have concerns about working conditions, try the U.S. Department of Labor (www.dol.gov) or the National Labor Relations Board (www.nlrb.gov).
  Tell legislators that all nurses in this country need whistleblower protection—now!

Implications for Practice: The decision to become a whistleblower can have far-reaching implications. If you decide to do so, proceed cautiously. Consider consulting first with other nursing, medical, and legal professionals.

CASE STUDY 5-2

Select an ethical issue of your choice in class, for example, should patients be given placebo medications?

Ask for one volunteer to give the reasons why patients should be given placebos and one volunteer to give the reasons why patients should not be given placebos.

Instruct your volunteers to consider all pertinent ethical theories and principles, any conflicts between them, any relationship to ethical codes, legal implications, people involved and impacted, and any relevant sociocultural, political, or religious aspects that may influence this ethical issue.

Each volunteer must state his or her position and references.

What pros were identified? What were the cons? Did any of the comments alter your own position on this question?

Developed with information from Ethical debates by L. Candela, S. R. Michael, and S. Mitchell, 2003. In *Nurse Educator, 28*(1), 37–39.

TABLE 5-9
ETHICAL PRINCIPLES AND RULES

Ethical Principle/Rule	Definition	Example
Beneficence	The duty to do good to others and to maintain a balance between benefits and harms.	• Provide all patients, including the terminally ill, with caring attention and information. • Become familiar with your state laws regarding organ donations. • Treat every patient with respect and courtesy.
Nonmaleficence	The principle of doing no harm.	• Always work within your scope of practice. • Never give information or perform duties when you are not qualified to do so. • Observe all safety rules and precautions. • Keep areas safe from hazards. • Perform procedures according to facility protocols. Never take shortcuts. • Ask an appropriate person about anything you are unsure of. • Keep your skills and education up to date.
Justice	The principle of fairness that is served when an individual is given that which he or she is due, owed, deserves, or can legitimately claim.	• Treat all patients equally, regardless of economic or social background. • Learn the local, state, and national laws and your facility's policies and procedures for handling and reporting suspected abuse.
Autonomy	Respect for an individual's right to self-determination; respect for individual liberty.	• Be sure that patients have consented to all treatments and procedures. • Become familiar with federal and state laws and facility policies dealing with privacy, e.g., HIPAA legislation.

(continues)

Table 5-9 *(continued)*

Ethical Principle/Rule	Definition	Example
		• Never release patient information of any kind unless there is a signed patient release. • Do not discuss patients with anyone who is not professionally involved in their care. • Protect the physical privacy of patients.
Fidelity	The principle of promise keeping; the duty to keep one's promise or word.	• Be sure that contracts have been completed. • Be very careful about what you say to patients. They may only hear the "good news."
Respect for others	The right of people to make their own decision.	• Provide all persons with information for decision making. • Avoid making paternalistic decisions for others.
Veracity	The obligation to tell the truth.	• Admit mistakes promptly. Offer to do whatever is necessary to correct them. • Refuse to participate in any form of fraud. • Give an "honest day's work" every day.
Advocacy	The obligation to look out or speak up for the rights of others.	• Provide patients with high quality, evidence-based care.

An Ethics Test. Health care practitioners may find that it is useful to run decision-making considerations through an ethics test when any doubt exists concerning an ethical issue. The ethics test presented here was used at the Center for Business Ethics at Bentley College (Buono & Bowditch, 2007) as part of ethical corporate training programs. Decision makers were taught to ask themselves:

- Is it right?
- Is it fair?

TABLE 5-10
CREATING AN ETHICAL WORKPLACE

Establishing an ethical and socially responsible workplace is not simply a matter of luck and common sense. Nurse managers can develop strategies and programs to enhance ethically and socially responsible attitudes. These may include:

1. Formal mechanisms for monitoring ethics, such as an ethics program or ethics committee
2. Written organizational codes of conduct
3. Widespread communication in the hospital to reinforce ethically and socially responsible behavior
4. Leadership by example: If people throughout the organization believe that behaving ethically is "in" and behaving unethically is "out," ethical behavior will prevail.
5. Encouraging confrontation about ethical deviations. Unethical behavior may be minimized if every employee confronts anyone seen behaving unethically.
6. Training programs in ethics and social responsibility, including messages about ethics from executives, classes on ethics at colleges, and exercises in ethics (DuBrin, 2008)
7. Instituting an ethics committee made up of representatives from nursing, medicine, administration, psychiatry, social work, nutritional services, and pharmacy, as well as an ethicist and patients and representatives from pastoral care. Additional persons may be invited on an as-needed basis. Ethical dilemmas may be referred to the ethics committee by anyone. This committee provides guidance to patients, families, and the health care team.
8. Refer to the ANA Code of Ethics for Nurses.

- Who gets hurt?
- Would you tell your child or young relative to do it?
- How does it smell? This question is based on a person's intuition and common sense.
- Would you be comfortable if the details of your decision were reported on the front page of your local newspaper or through your hospital's e-mail system?

RISK MANAGEMENT PROGRAMS

Risk management programs in health care organizations are designed to identify and correct system problems that contribute to errors in patient care or to employee injury. The emphasis in risk management programs is on quality improvement and protection of the organization from financial liability. Organizations usually have reporting and tracking forms that record incidents that may lead to financial liability for the organization. Risk management will assist in identifying and correcting the underlying problem that may have led to an incident, such as faulty equipment, staffing or delegation concerns, or the need for better orientation for employees. Once a system problem is identified, the Risk Management Department may develop strategies and educational programs for health care staff to address the problem.

The Risk Management Department may also investigate and record information surrounding a patient or employee incident that may result in a lawsuit. This helps personnel remember critical factors if called to testify at a later time. The nurse should notify the Risk Management Department of all reportable incidents and complete all Risk Management and/or Incident Report forms as mandated by institutional policies and procedures. Note that employee complaints of harassment or discrimination can expose the institution to significant liability and should promptly be reported to supervisors and the Risk Management Department, to Human Resources, or another department as specified in the institution's policies. The Risk Management Department staff also participate on key hospital committees, such as the Patient Safety Committee, Environment of Care Committee, Pharmacy and Nursing Committee, Ethics Committee, and other hospital committees that work on proactive programs to reduce risks (Martin, Cain, & Priest, 2008). See Table 5-11 for a checklist of actions to decrease the risk of liability.

TABLE 5-11
CHECKLIST OF ACTIONS TO DECREASE LIABILITY
Nursing
• Use the National Council of State Boards of Nursing (NCSBN) Delegation Decision-Making Tree or your organization's delegation grid to make safe delegation decisions.   • Delegate patient care based on patients' needs, staff competency and skill, and the documented education, skill, and experience of licensed and unlicensed personnel.

(continues)

Table 5-11 *(continued)*

- Develop a professional, assertive communication style with health care providers to assist you with meeting patient care goals. Identify realistic, attainable outcome standards to use to identify completion of any task that is delegated. Make frequent walking rounds to assure quality patient outcomes after delegation.
- Treat all patients and their families with kindness and respect.
- Take appropriate actions to meet the patients' nursing needs.
- Communicate with your patients and keep them informed.
- Communicate the patient's name, room number, and expectations for staff before, during, and after duty performance in a pleasant, direct, and concise manner when delegating patient care.
- Acknowledge unfortunate incidents and express concern about these events without either taking the blame, blaming others, or reacting defensively.
- Promptly report any concern regarding the quality of care, including the lack of resources with which to provide care, faulty equipment, staffing concerns, medication concerns, orientation or education concerns, complaints of discrimination or harassment, and patient or family complaints to a nursing administration representative.
- Follow evidence-based standards of care and the facility's policy and procedure for administering care and reporting incidents. Document the reason for any omission or deviation from the standards.
- Maintain current professional standards of care and clinical competency. Acknowledge your limitations. If you do not know how to do something, ask for help.
- Assume personal responsibility to develop professional educational certifications and clinical expertise.
- Encourage the development of clearly written and/or computerized orders from all health care providers.
- Chart and time your observations immediately, while facts are still fresh in your mind.
- Document the time of nursing actions and changes in conditions requiring notification of the health care provider. Include the response of the provider. Use the chain of command at your organization to report any concerns. Use SBARR as a guide.
- Complete incident reports immediately after incidents occur. Discuss critical factors with the risk manager to increase your retention of the facts.
- Follow professional guidelines for safe transfer of all patients both inside and outside the organization.

(continues)

Table 5-11 *(continued)*

Organizational

- Follow professional standards for education, licensure, and competency in all hiring decisions, orientation, and ongoing continuing education programs.
- Have clear job descriptions and ongoing licensing and credentialing policies for health care providers, LPN/LVNs, nursing assistive personnel (NAP), and other health care staff. The organization must ensure that all staff are safe, competent practitioners before assigning them to patient care. Orient all staff to each other's roles and job descriptions.
- Provide standards for ongoing supervision and periodic licensure/competency verification and evaluation of all staff.
- Provide access to professional health care standards, policies, procedures, library, and medication information with unit availability and efficient Internet access.
- Have clear policies and procedures for delegation and chain-of-command reporting lines for all staff from RN to charge nurse to nurse manager to nurse executive and, as appropriate, to risk management, the hospital ethics committee, the hospital administrator, medical practitioners, the chief of the medical staff, the board of directors, the State Licensing Board for Nursing and Medicine, and the Accreditation Agency.
- Provide administrative support for supervisors and staff who delegate, assign, monitor, and evaluate patient care.
- Clarify health care provider accountability; for example, if the medical practitioner delegates a nursing task to NAP, the medical practitioner is responsible for monitoring that care delivery. This must be spelled out in hospital policy. If the RN notes that the NAP is doing something incorrectly, the RN has a duty to intervene and to notify the ordering practitioner of the incident. The RN always has an independent responsibility to protect patient safety. Blindly relying on another nursing or medical practitioner is not permissible for the RN.
- Provide standards for regular RN evaluation of NAP and LPN/LVNs and reinforce the need for NAP and LPN/LVN accountability to RN. RNs must delegate and supervise. They cannot abdicate this professional responsibility.
- Develop physical, mental, and verbal "No Abuse" policy to be followed by all professional and nonprofessional health care staff.
- Consider applying for magnet status for your facility. This status is awarded by the American Nurses Credentialing Center to Hospitals that have worked to improve nursing care, including the empowering of nursing decision making and delegation in clinical practice.

(continues)

Table 5-11 *(continued)*

- Consider a shared governance model of nursing practice to empower nursing decision making and delegation in clinical practice.
- Monitor patient outcomes, including nurse-sensitive outcomes; staffing ratios; and other clinical, financial, and organizational quality indicators.
- Develop ongoing clinical quality improvement practices.
- Maintain ongoing monitoring of incident reports, sentinel events, and other elements of risk management and performance improvement of the process and outcome of patient care.
- Develop systematic, error-proof systems for medication administration that ensure the six "rights" of medication administration, that is, the right patient, right medication, right dose, right time, right route, and right documentation. Include computerized order entry.
- Provide documentation of routine maintenance for all patient care equipment.
- Attain Joint Commission Patient Safety Goals, 2010.
- Avoid problems and monitor the Medicare-Medicaid, Do Not Pay List (Medicare's Do Not Pay List, 2008), e.g., do not give patients the wrong type of blood.

KEEP YOUR PATIENTS SAFE 5-3

You are the only RN assigned to give 9 a.m. medications on a 52-bed nursing home unit. To avoid being classified as a drug error according to the organization's policy and usual nursing practice, administration of the medications must occur within 45 minutes of the ordered time. Also, nursing practice mandates that you verify the six "rights": the right drug, the right dose, the right patient, the right time, the right route, and the right documentation.

What problems are there with this assignment? What would you do?

REAL WORLD INTERVIEW

The role of risk management in the health care environment is that of recognition, evaluation, and treatment of risks inherent in the organization. The goal of risk management is improving the quality of care provided by the organization while at the same time protecting its financial integrity. Risk management, while coordinated at a certain level of the organization, is not simply a one-department responsibility, but rather is the responsibility of each employee of the organization.

(continues)

Real World Interview *(continued)*

New graduates in nursing need to understand that in today's competitive health care environment, it is important that each practitioner look for ways to reduce the risks inherent in the delivery of health care. At a time when hospitals are receiving less and less reimbursement, our patients and consumers are demanding higher and higher quality of care.

Health care is at a crossroads, similar to the one that faced private industry during the 1970s. Our customers are demanding that we provide a safe environment and that we consistently strive for continuous quality improvement.

An incident report is a commonly used form that documents a variance from normal protocol or hospital procedures. It is not meant to place blame on an individual practitioner or department. It is used strictly to document the facts surrounding an event so the health care processes can be improved. Thus, the nurse should complete an incident report when any variance from a policy or a procedure is noticed.

When risk management receives the incident reports, they are logged into our database, and monthly reports are forwarded to nurse mangers for follow-up and education with their staff.

Incident reports and the subsequent risk management department actions are generally reactive, but we also do proactive/preventive interventions in the health care setting. These include the following:
1. Education of students completing their senior year of study in nursing
2. Participation on patient safety, environment of care, pharmacy, nursing, and other hospital committees, which work on proactive programs to reduce risks
3. Facilitation of the slips and falls task force to reduce our patients' fall risk
4. Education of new nurses and physicians on principles of risk management

Harriet Percy, RN
Risk Manager
New Orleans, Louisiana

MALPRACTICE/PROFESSIONAL LIABILITY INSURANCE

Nurses often wonder if they should carry their own malpractice insurance. Nurses may think their actions are adequately covered by the employer's liability insurance, but this is not necessarily so. While the organization's insurance company almost always pays malpractice awards, insurance contracts often have provisions that allow them to refuse payment if the insured intentionally injures another party (Pozza, 2003). Also, if in giving care, the nurse fails to comply with the organization's policies and procedures, the organization may deny the nurse a defense, claiming that because of the nurse's failure to follow organizational policy the nurse was not acting as an employee at that time. Nurses are also being named individually as defendants in malpractice suits more frequently than was the case in the past, although organizations are often a plaintiff's primary target because they typically have deeper pockets than individual practitioners (Pozza, 2003). It is advantageous for the nurse to be assured of a defense independent of that of his or her employer. Professional liability insurance provides that assurance and pays for an attorney to defend the nurse in a malpractice lawsuit.

Note that in the event that an unaffiliated nurse, such as an agency per diem nurse, is held individually liable for a judgment, the nurse's personal insurance carrier will be responsible for paying the verdict rendered against the nurse. An unaffiliated, uninsured nurse could be forced to pay for her own defense and be financially responsible for any judgments rendered against her (Pozza, 2003).

In making the decision whether to obtain separate insurance, a nurse should consider the value of his or her personal assets. A nurse should also consider the laws of the state in which he or she practices regarding those assets that are exempt from being seized to satisfy civil monetary judgments. Generally, one home and one automobile are exempt from seizure (Pozza, 2003).

NURSING RISK IN LITIGATION

Nurses may be sued individually for damages resulting from their negligent acts.[13, 15, 16, 18, 23, 30, 38, 44] However, often a plaintiff will name the nurse's employer as a defendant instead of, or in addition to, suing the nurse individually. In other words, a hospital, nursing home, or clinic is often held legally responsible for the damages caused by the negligence of its nurses. It is well-established law throughout the United States that "a master is subject to liability for the torts of his servants committed while acting in the scope of employment."[50] This law is called Respondeat Superior. It is set out in the Restatement of the Law of Agency. The Restatement sets forth principles of common law that are generally accepted in all courts throughout the country. Respondeat Superior is one such law.

A plaintiff may also sue the hospital, nursing home, or health clinic for its direct negligence. For example, nursing homes have been sued for failing to adequately train and supervise personnel.[8, 19, 24, 34] Hospitals have been sued for allowing unlicensed personnel to administer medications[34] and for failing to provide appropriate laboratory services to patients.[23] Hospitals may also be held legally responsible for failing to maintain appropriate policies and procedures regarding staffing, quality assurance, and chain of command (Pozza, 2003).

In many malpractice cases involving hospitals, the health care providers involved are also named individually.[1, 3, 6, 7, 11, 12, 13, 21, 24, 26, 28, 33, 34, 37, 40, 41, 43] Customarily, plaintiffs in medical malpractice cases name a combination of health care providers as defendants. It is common for some or all of the defendants to settle the cases before they reach the trial phase. However, in the event that a case proceeds to trial, a jury may find that none, some, or all of the defendants were negligent in their care and treatment of the plaintiff. A jury may determine that the nursing care was appropriate, but the medical treatment was substandard. Likewise, a jury could hold that the health care provider rendered appropriate care, but the nurses' conduct fell below the standard of care. Additionally, a recent trend in malpractice litigation is to name the Health Maintenance Organization (HMO) as a defendant as well. For example, the Illinois Supreme Court recently held that an HMO could be liable under theories of apparent authority, respondeat superior, direct corporate negligence, breach of contract, and breach of warranty[48] (Pozza, 2003).

Common Monetary Awards.   Many health care malpractice cases are dismissed or settled prior to trial. In those cases that do reach the trial stage, jury verdicts are unpredictable and awards can vary dramatically. For instance, juries awarded the following for the listed injuries:

- Brachial plexus injury ($13.3 million)[6]
- Wrongful death—pulmonary embolism ($5 million)[1]
- Microcephaly in newborn ($17 million)[11]
- Vision loss ($8 million)[13]
- Arterial impairment ($260,000)[51]

A jury may award the plaintiff both compensatory and punitive damages. Compensatory damages are awarded to compensate the plaintiff for his or her injuries. Compensatory damages include damages for both economic losses (medical expenses, lost wages, lost earning capacity) and non-economic losses (pain and suffering).

Punitive damages are not intended to compensate the plaintiff for any loss. Rather, punitive damages are intended to punish the defendant for acting with "recklessness, malice or deceit."[54] Punitive damage awards are particularly common in cases involving nursing homes. For example, a Texas jury awarded the family of a nursing home resident $90 million in punitive damages for gross negligence that caused the resident to develop pressure ulcers and contractures[49] (Pozza, 2003).

Selected Monetary Liability Limits. Since 1970, at least 30 states have enacted legislation capping the monetary damages plaintiffs can recover in a lawsuit.[53] Currently, there are as many different cap schemes as states that employ them. Some states cap the amount that a plaintiff may receive for punitive damages.

Other states employ a flat dollar cap. These states limit the total monetary amount the plaintiff may recover in both compensatory and punitive damages in any malpractice action.

A plaintiff may claim he or she is entitled to damages in excess of the applicable cap. Jurors are customarily not informed of the caps applicable in their states. Therefore, it is common for a jury's award to exceed the state's cap on damages. In the event that a jury awards a plaintiff damages in excess of a statutory cap, the judge will reduce the jury's award to the cap (Pozza, 2003).

Other Legal Risks for the Nurse/Practitioner/Hospital. In addition to increased insurance premiums, health care providers have much at stake when named as defendants in malpractice cases. Health care providers are required to report adverse verdicts and settlements to the National Practitioner's Data Bank. The National Practitioner's Data Bank was established through the Health Care Quality Improvement Act of 1986. The federal regulations regarding the Data Bank can be found in 45 Code of Federal Regulations (CFR) Part 60. Significant awards against health care providers or numerous malpractice payments by health care providers can affect the health care providers licensure or ability to gain privileges to practice at certain hospitals and health care entities. Failure to report malpractice payments to the Data Bank can result in civil monetary penalties. The U.S. Department of Health and Human Services, Office of the Inspector General, may impose a civil "monetary" penalty of up to $11,000 for each violation.

Federal and state statutes and regulations prescribe nursing standards of care. See the Code of Federal Regulations Title 42-Public Health and Title 45-Public Welfare. See also U.S. Code Title 42-Public Health and Welfare. Every jurisdiction that licenses nurses has a nurse practice act.[52] In addition to instructing nurses on the definition of the standard of care for that jurisdiction, the nurse practice act mandates strict rules for reporting and disciplining nurses who violate the standard. Likewise, state boards of nursing may take action to suspend or revoke the licenses of nurses determined by the board to have violated the standard of care. Private entities, such as the Joint Commission (JC), and professional organizations, such as the American Nurses Association (ANA), promulgate their own rules of conduct that serve as guidelines for acceptable nursing care (Pozza, 2003).

EVIDENCE FROM THE LITERATURE

Citation: Jha, A. K., Doolan, D., Grandt, D., Scott, T., & Bates, D. W. (2008). The use of health information technology in seven nations. *International Journal of Medical Informatics, 24*(Jul), 254–262.

Discussion: The authors assessed the state of health information technology (HIT) adoption and use in seven industrialized nations. They used a combination of literature review, as well as interviews with experts in individual nations, to determine the use of key information technologies. They examined the rate of electronic health record (EHR) use in ambulatory care and hospital settings, along with current activities in health information exchange (HIE) in seven countries: the United States (U.S.), Canada, United Kingdom (UK), Germany, Netherlands, Australia, and New Zealand (NZ). Four nations (the UK, Netherlands, Australia, and NZ) had nearly universal use of EHRs among general practitioners (each nation was >90%), and Germany was moving forward (ranged from 40%–80%). The U.S. and Canada had a minority of ambulatory care physicians who used EHRs consistently ranged from 10%–30%. While there are no high-quality data for the hospital setting from any of the nations the authors examined, evidence suggests that only a small fraction of hospitals (<10%) in any single country had the key components of an EHR. HIE efforts were a high priority in all seven nations, but early efforts have revealed varying degrees of active clinical data exchange.

Implications for Practice: Increased efforts will be needed if interoperable EHRs are soon to become universally available and used in these seven nations. Nurses and other practitioners in these nations must be part of the solution to making the EHR universally used and available.

NURSE-ATTORNEY RELATIONSHIP IN A LAWSUIT

In spite of the nurse's best intentions, a nurse may be named as a defendant in a lawsuit and need to retain the services of an attorney. LaDuke (2000) makes the following suggestions for consulting and collaborating with an attorney:

1. Retain a legal specialist. Generalist lawyers are competent to handle many matters, but professional malpractice, professional disciplinary proceedings, and employment disputes are best handled by specialists in those areas.

2. Be attentive. Read the documents the attorney produces, and travel to court proceedings to observe the attorney's performance.

3. Notify your insurance carrier as soon as you are aware of any real or potential liability issue. Inform your agent about the status of your case every few months, even if it's unchanged.

4. Keep costs sensible. Your attorney should explain initially how the fee will be computed and how you will be billed. The attorney may require you to pay a retainer fee.

5. Keep informed. The attorney should address your questions and concerns promptly. You are entitled to be kept informed about the status of your case. You are entitled to copies of all correspondence, legal briefs, and other documents.

6. Examine all writing. Your attorney needs to explain all facts and options. Examine all relevant documents, and do not hesitate to make corrections in the same way you would correct a medical record by drawing a line through the incorrect or misleading information, writing in the correction, and signing your initials after it.

7. Set your own course. Insist on a collaborative relationship with your attorney for the duration of your case.

 ## REVIEW QUESTIONS

1. Jose, RN, discussed a patient with the patient's employer. This invasion of privacy is an example of which of the following? Commission of:
   A. A tort
   B. An administrative law violation
   C. A Good Samaritan Law violation
   D. A criminal law violation

2. Inez, RN, did not put the bed siderails up on a confused patient. The patient fell and was injured. When there is a connection between the nurse omitting a duty and the damages occurring to a patient, this is an example of which of the following?
   A. Breach of duty
   B. Duty
   C. Causation
   D. Damages

3. Select the most appropriate documentation example below.
   A. Patient found covered in stool. The night nurses were too busy to change the bed.
   B. The patient fell because we are short of staff.
   C. The patient's family is difficult and argumentative.
   D. Dr. M. Bresley notified through the medical exchange at 0610 of patient's complaints of difficulty breathing. Orders received for oxygen and ABGs.

4. You call the surgeon for your new postoperative patient, who is bleeding excessively. The patient's blood pressure has decreased by 20 mm Hg, and his pulse rate has increased by 20 beats over the past hour. The surgeon's response to this information is, "Why did you wake me up at 2 a.m. for this? I am hanging up, as I expect a postoperative patient to be oozing from the operative site and these changes are not significant. Just watch him." You are quite concerned about your patient. What will you do next?
   A. Go to the nursing station and complain to the other nurses about how rude the surgeon was on the phone.
   B. Document and quote the surgeon's response in your nurse's notes.
   C. Inform the surgeon that you do not agree with continuing to just observe this patient and that you are going to initiate the chain of command.
   D. Tell the family what the surgeon said.

5. An 80-year-old male who lives with his son is brought to your unit because "he isn't acting right." On physical examination, you note that the patient is malnourished, noncommunicative, and has poor hygiene. When asking the patient some questions, he avoids eye contact and does not respond. The son is answering questions for the patient and refuses to leave the room. You suspect elder abuse. Choose the most appropriate documentation of the situation.
   A. The patient is very thin and does not make eye contact with the nursing or medical staff. It is obvious that he has been abused and neglected by his family.
   B. The patient is a thin elderly male who presents to the unit wearing clothing that is soiled. He does not make eye contact with the staff or answer our questions. Social services notified.
   C. It appears that the patient's son manipulates his father by refusing to let his father answer any questions. We suspect elder abuse.
   D. The patient's son states that the patient "isn't acting right." The patient does not answer questions from the staff due to his abuse.

6. The nurse is given a written order by a health care provider to administer an unusually large dose of pain medicine to a patient. In this situation, which of the following is an appropriate nursing action?
   A. Administer the medication because it was ordered by a health care provider.
   B. Refuse to administer the medication, and move on to another patient.
   C. Speak with the health care provider about your concerns, and clarify whether the medication dose is accurate.
   D. Select a dose that you feel comfortable with, and administer that dose.

7. A health care provider has ordered you to discharge Mr. Jones from the hospital, despite a new temperature of 102.0°F (38.8°C). The provider refuses to talk with you about the patient. In this situation, which of the following is an appropriate nursing action?
   A. Administer an antipyretic medication and discharge the patient.
   B. Discharge the patient with instructions to call 911 if he has any problems.
   C. Do not discharge the patient until you have discussed the matter with your nursing manager and are satisfied regarding patient safety.
   D. Discharge the patient and tell the patient to take Tylenol when he gets home.

8. A health care provider has issued a Do Not Attempt to Resuscitate (DNAR) order for your patient, a 55-year-old man with cancer. You spoke with the patient this morning, and he clearly wishes to be resuscitated in the event that he stops breathing. What is the most appropriate course of action?
   A. Ignore the patient's wishes because the health care provider ordered the DNAR.
   B. Consult your hospital's policies and procedures, speak to the health care provider, and discuss the matter with your nurse manager.
   C. Attempt to talk the patient into agreeing to the DNAR.
   D. Contact the medical licensing board to complain about the health care provider.

9. The Health Insurance Portability and Accountability Act (HIPAA) protects which of the following?
   A. A patient's right to be insured, regardless of employment status or ability to pay
   B. The confidentiality of certain protected health information
   C. The nurse's right to health insurance
   D. The hospital's right to disclose protected health information

10. Which of the following elements is not necessary for a nurse to be found negligent in a court of law?
    A. A duty or obligation for the nurse to act in a particular way
    B. A breach of that duty or obligation
    C. The nurse's intention to be negligent
    D. Physical, emotional, or financial harm to the patient

11. You are a new nurse working on a medical-surgical unit. One of your patients, an elderly woman, has an advance directive that requests that no CPR be done in the event that she stops breathing. One day she

stops breathing, and someone on your unit calls a "code" and begins resuscitative efforts. You go along with the team and help to resuscitate the patient. She regains a pulse, but never regains consciousness. She is now ventilator-dependent, and her family is very angry with you and the staff. Which of the following is a potential legal action you will face?

A. Violation of patient privacy
B. Battery
C. Criminal recklessness
D. Revoked nursing license

12. Which of the following is not an essential element of a Good Samaritan Law?

A. The care is rendered in an emergency situation.
B. The health care worker is rendering care without pay.
C. The health care worker is concerned about the safety of the victims.
D. The care provided did not recklessly or intentionally cause injury or harm to the injured party.

APPLY YOUR SKILLS

1. Talk to the Risk Manager at the hospital where you have your clinical assignments. Ask him to comment about the hospital committees on which he serves. How do the Risk Management Department and other hospital committees work to decrease hospital liability and improve patient care?

2. Identify the various ways in which nurses you observe in your clinical rotations discuss orders and treatments with health care providers. How do nurses address incorrect or questionable medication orders? Talk with nurses you encounter about how they handle these situations.

3. Research the various companies that offer nursing malpractice insurance, and determine the cost and coverage associated with a nursing malpractice policy. Go to an Internet search engine, such as www.google.com. Search for "Nursing Malpractice Insurance." What did you find? Note the Nursing Service Organization (NSO) Web site at www.nso.com. Recent legal cases are reported there.

4. It is important to monitor your state nurse practice act. See the list of Web sites provided in Table 5-14.

TABLE 5-14
NURSE PRACTICE ACTS

Note your individual State Board of Nursing Web site: Go to your state link and search for "State Board of Nursing."

Alabama: http://www.abn.state.al.us
Alaska: http://www.dced.state.ak.us
Arizona: http://www.azboardofnursing.org
Arkansas: http://www.state.ar.us
California RN: http://www.rn.ca.gov
California VN: http://www.bvnpt.ca.gov
Colorado: http://www.dora.state.co.us
Connecticut: http://www.state.ct.us
Florida: http://www.doh.state.fl.us
Georgia PN: http://www.sos.state.ga.us
Hawaii: http://www.state.hi.us
Idaho: http://www.state.id.us
Illinois: http://www.dpr.state.il.us
Indiana: http://www.state.in.us
Iowa: http://www.state.ia.us
Kansas: http://www.ksbn.org
Kentucky: http://www.kbn.state.ky.us
Louisiana PN: http://www.lsbpne.com
Louisiana RN: http://www.lsbn.state.la.us
Maine: http://www.state.me.us
Maryland: http://dhmh1d.dhmh.state.md.us
Massachusetts: http://www.state.ma.us
Michigan: http://www.cis.state.mi.us
Minnesota: http://www.nursingboard.state.mn.us
Mississippi: http://www.msbn.state.ms.us
Missouri: http://www.ecodev.state.mo.us
Montana: http://www.com.state.mt.us
Nebraska: http://www.hhs.state.ne.us
Nevada: http://www.nursingboard.state.nv.us
New Hampshire: http://www.state.nh.us
New Jersey: http://www.state.nj.us
New Mexico: http://www.state.nm.us
New York: http://www.nysed.gov
North Carolina: http://www.ncbon.com
North Dakota: http://www.ndbon.org
Ohio: http://www.state.oh.us
Oregon: http://www.osbn.state.or.us
Pennsylvania: http://www.dos.state.pa.us
Rhode Island: http://www.health.state.ri.us
South Carolina: http://www.llr.state.sc.us
South Dakota: http://www.state.sd.us
Tennessee: http://health.state.tn.us
Texas RN: http://www.bne.state.tx.us

(continues)

Table 5-14 *(continued)*

Texas VN: http://www.bvne.state.tx.us
Utah: http://www.commerce.state.ut.us
Vermont: http://vtprofessionals.org
Virginia: http://www.dhp.state.va.us
Washington: http://www.doh.wa.gov
West Virginia PN: http://www.lpnboard.state.wv.us
West Virginia RN: http://www.state.wv.us
Wisconsin: http://www.drl.state.wi.us
Wyoming: http://nursing.state.wy.us

EXPLORING THE WEB

1. Visit this site for state and federal laws regulating hospitals:
   www.findlaw.com

2. Find a copy of the ANA Code of Ethics at:
   www.nursingworld.org

3. Check this site for ANA papers:
   www.nursingworld.org

   Note various papers on the role of the nurse. Also note information about magnet hospitals and risk management that can be accessed through this site. ANA membership is required to access some papers.

4. Note the information available at:
   www.ncsbn.org

5. The Code of Federal Regulations is available at the United States Government Printing Office Web site:
   www.gpo.gov

6. The United States Code is available at the Office of the Law Revision Counsel Web site:
   http://uscode.house.gov

7. Find legal research at the Law and Policy Institutions Guide:
   www.lpig.org

8. Consider the information you can find at these sites:
   www.westlaw.com
   www.lexis.com
   www.aslme.com
   www.jointcommission.org
   www.cms.hhs.gov

9. Go to this site to find malpractice information for your state:
   www.mcandl.com

10. You have a patient who is to be transferred to a nursing home for recuperation. Where can you tell the family to look to evaluate the local nursing homes regarding their adherence to the federal regulations for nursing homes? Suggest:
www.medicare.gov

11. Visit the Medical Liability Monitor at:
www.medicalliabilitymonitor.com

    Also visit this site:
    http://aspe.hhs.gov
    What did you find there?

12. Go to www.google.com, and type in "living wills" and "power of attorney." What did you find there?

REFERENCES

Adams, S. (2004). HIPAA patient confidentiality requirements. *Journal of Emergency Nursing, 30*(1), 70.

American Nurses Association (ANA). (2001a). *Code of ethics.* Silver Spring, MD: Author.

American Nurses Association (ANA). (2001b). *Code of Ethics for Nurses.* Retrieved March 1, 2010, from http://nursingworld.org/MainMenuCategories/EthicsStandards/CodeofEthicsforNurses.aspx

Americans with Disabilities Act (ADA). (1990). Retrieved March 14, 2010, from www.ada.gov/pubs/ada.htm

Austin, S. (2006). Seven legal tips for safe nursing practice. *Nursing, 38*(3), 34–39, quiz 39-40.

Berdyck v. Shinde, 613 N.E. 2d 1014, 1024. (1993).

Buono, A. F., & Bowditch, J. L. (2007). *Primer on organizational behavior.* New York, NY: Wiley.

Candela, L., Michael, S. R., & Mitchell, S. (2003). Ethical debates. *Nurse Educator, 28*(1), 37–39.

Code of Federal Regulations. (n.d.). Retrieved March 1, 2010, from www.gpoaccess.gov/CFR

Croke, E. M. (2003). Nurses, negligence, and malpractice. *American Journal of Nursing, 103*(9), 54–64.

Cruzan v. Director, Missouri Department of Health, 110 S. Ct. 2841. (1990).

DeLaune, S. C., & Ladner, P. K. (2011). *Fundamentals of nursing* (4th ed.). Clifton Park, NY: Delmar Cengage Learning.

DuBrin, A. J. (2008). *Essentials of management.* Clifton Park, NY: Delmar Cengage Learning.

Electronic health record. (2008). In *Wikipedia.* Retrieved October 2, 2008, from http:// en.wikipedia.org/wiki/electronic_health_records_over_paper_records

Frank-Stromborg, M. (2004). They're real and they're here: The new federally regulated privacy rules under HIPAA. *Dermatology Nursing, 16*(1), 13–24.

Hellquist, K., & Spector, N. (2004). A primer: The national council of state boards of nursing nurse licensure compact. *Journal of Nursing Administration's Healthcare Law, Ethics, and Regulation, 6*(4), 86–89.

Jha, A. K., Doolan, D., Grandt, D., Scott, T., & Bates, D. W. (2008). The use of health information technology in seven nations. *International Journal of Medical Informatics, 24*(Jul), 254–262.

LaDuke, S. (2000). What should you expect from your attorney? *Nursing Management, 31*(1), 10.

Martin, J., Cain, K., & Priest, C. S. (2008). In P. Kelly (Ed.), *Nursing leadership & management* (2nd ed.). Clifton Park, NY: Delmar Cengage Learning.

Medicare's Do Not Pay List, Medicare. (2008). Retrieved March 1, 2010, from www.medicare-medicaid.com

Murphy v. United Parcel Service, 527 U.S. 516. (1999).

National Council of State Boards of Nursing. (1997). *Delegation decision-making tree.* Retrieved October 2, 2008, from www.ncsbn.org/887. htm?search-text=delegation+decision+making+tree&select=%23

National Practitioner Data Bank (NPDB). (n.d.). *Healthcare Integrity and Protection Data Bank.* Retrieved March 1, 2010, from www.npdb-hipdb.hrsa.gov

Nurse Licensure Compact, National Council of the State Boards of Nursing. (n. d.). Retrieved March 1, 2010, from www.ncsbn.org/158.htm

Occupational Safety & Health Administration (OSHA). (n.d.). *U.S. Department of Labor.* Retrieved October 2, 2010, from www.osha.gov

Odom v. State Department of Health and Hospitals, 322 So. 2d 91 (La. App. 1999).

Pozza, R. (2003). *Legal aspects of nursing.* Unpublished Manuscript. Austin, TX.

Roe v. Wade, 410 U.S. 133. (1973).

Shay, E. F. (2005). Legal barriers to electronic health records. *Physician News Digest.* Retrieved March 1, 2010, from www.physiciansnews.com/law/505.html

Sutton v. United Airlines, 527 U.S. 471. (1999).

The Civil Rights Act of 1964. (1964). Retrieved March 1, 2010, from www.archives.gov/education/lessons/civil-rights-act

The 'Lectric Law Library's Lexicon On Tort. (2008). Retrieved March 1, 2010, from www.lectlaw.com/def2/t032.htm

Vonfrolio, L. G. (2006, October). Blow the whistle? *RN, 69*(10), 60.

Webb v. Tulane Medical Center Hospital, 700 So. 2d 1141, 1145 (La. App. 1997).

SUGGESTED READINGS

Erlen, J. (2004). HIPAA: Clinical and ethical considerations for nurses. *Orthopaedic Nursing, 23*(6), 410–413.

Kay Hall, J. (2004). After Schiavo: Next issue for nursing ethics. *Journal of Nursing Administration's Healthcare Law, Ethics, and Regulation, 7*(3), 94–98.

Priest, C. (2005). Held liable. *Reflections on Nursing Leadership, 31*(1), 20–22, 36.

Ziel, S. (2004). Guard against HIPAA violations. *Nursing Management, 35*(4), 26–27.

CASE REFERENCES

1. Martinelli v. Lifemark Hosps. of Fla., Inc., Fla., Dade County Cir. Ct., No. 99-14491 CA 05, Mar. 1, 2001. 16 *ATLA* PNLR 111, July 2001.

2. Doe v. Roe Hosp., Ohio, Cuyahoga County C.C.P., confidential docket number, Feb. 2001. 16 *PNLR* 113, July 2001.

3. Montalvo v. Mercy Hosp., Tex., Webb County 111th Jud. Dist. Ct., No. 98-CVQ-01126-D2, Aug. 4, 2000. 16 *PNLR* 116, July 2001.

4. Doe v. Roe, confidential state, court, and docket number, Dec. 2000. 16 *PNLR* 117, July 2001.

5. Fuqua v. Horizon/CMS Healthcare Corp., U.S. Dist. Ct., N.D. Tex., No. 4-98-CV-1087-Y, Feb. 14, 2001. 16 *PNLR* 117, July 2001.

6. Stonieczny v. Gardner, Ill., Cook County Cir. Ct., No. 98 L 04578, May 29, 2001. 16 *PNLR* 131, Sept. 2001.

7. Doe v. Roe, N.C., confidential court and docket number, Dec. 4, 2000. 16 *PNLR* 137, Sept. 2001.

8. Nash v. Compton Mgmt., Inc., Ark., Cross County Cir. Ct., No. CIV-99-34, June 7, 2001. 16 *PNLR* 137, Sept. 2001.

9. Copeland v. Dallas Home for Jewish Aged, Inc., Tex., Dallas County 134th Jud. Dist. Ct., No. 98-04690, May 21, 2001. 16 *PNLR* 138, Sept. 2001.

10. Doe v. Kimberly QualityCare, Inc., Ariz., Maricopa County Super. Ct., No. CV-96-10499, June 1, 2001. 16 *PNLR* 149, Oct. 2001.

11. Diver v. Gingo, Ohio, Cuyahoga County C.C.P., No. 305538, Jan. 2001. 16 *PNLR* 152, Oct. 2001.

12. Williams v. Hospital Auth. of Valdosta, U.S. Dist. Ct., M.D. Ga., No. 7:98-CV-79(WDO), Dec. 23, 2000. 16 *PNLR* 152, Oct. 2001.

13. Schwab v. Kamat, N.Y., Onondaga County Sup. Ct., No. 97-887, June 8, 2001. 16 *PNLR* 154, Oct. 2001.

14. Furman v. San Pedro Peninsula Hosp., Cal., Los Angeles County Super. Ct., No. NC025678, Feb. 28, 2001. 16 *PNLR* 154, Oct. 2001.

15. Marshal v. Methodist Healthcare Jackson Hosp., Miss., Hinds County Cir. Ct., No. 251-99-000984CIV, Jan. 23, 2001. 16 *PNLR* 174, Nov. 2001.

16. Lewis v. Physicians Ins. Co. of Wis., 627 N.W.2d 484. 16 *PNLR* 175, Nov. 2001.

17. Doe v. Roe Med. Group, Ohio, Richland County C.C.P., confidential docket no., Mar. 20, 2001. 16 *PNLR* 176, Nov. 2001.

18. Doe v. Roe, confidential court and docket no., Apr. 2001. 16 *PNLR* 177, Nov. 2001.

19. Sauer v. Advocat, Inc., Ark., Polk County Cir. Ct., No. CIV-2000-5, June 22, 2001. 16 *PNLR* 179, Nov. 2001.

20. Johnson v. Commonwealth of Virginia, Va., Stafford County Cir. Ct., No. 99191, Apr. 2001. 16 *PNLR* 197, Dec. 2001.

21. Couch v. St. Luke's Med. Ctr. RMC, Idaho, Ada County Dist. Ct., Nos. 9900289D, 99000358D, May 2001. 16 *PNLR* 197, Dec. 2001.

22. Doe v. United States, confidential court and docket no., 2001. 16 *PNLR* 200, Dec. 2001.

23. Urgent v. Government of the Virgin Islands, U.S.V.I., V.I. Territorial Ct. St. Croix Div., No. 607/1998, Sept. 13, 2001. 17 *PNLR* 8, Feb. 2002.

24. Johns v. Franciscan Health Sys. W., Wash., King County Super. Ct., No. 99-2-04211-5KNT, Oct. 30, 2001. 17 *PNLR* 9, Feb. 2002.

25. Doe v. Sibley Hosp., D.C., D.C. Super. Ct., No. 983387, Aug. 16, 2001. 17 *PNLR* 9, Feb. 2002.

26. Chichy v. Ghate, Pa., Indiana County C.C.P., No. 11048 CD 1997, June 25, 2001. 17 *PNLR* 10, Feb. 2002.

27. Arledge v. Oak Grove Nursing Home, Inc., Tex., Jefferson County 58th Jud. Dist. Ct., No. A162668, Sept. 18, 2001. 17 *PNLR* 11, Feb. 2002.

28. Lee v. Chen, Ill., Cook County Cir. Ct., No. 95 L 2796, Sept. 27, 2001. 17 *PNLR* 28, Mar. 2002.

29. Graham v. Forrest Gen. Hosp., Miss., Forrest County Cir. Ct., No. CI00-0165, June 12, 2001. 17 *PNLR* 31, Mar. 2002.

30. Lavalis v. Copperas Cove L.L.C., Tex., Bell County 146th Jud. Dist. Ct., No. 183,293-B, Dec. 27, 2001. 17 *PNLR* 32, Mar. 2002.

31. Doe v. Roe Nursing Home, U.S. Dist. Ct., D. Kan., No. 99-1474 WEB, Aug. 2001. 17 *PNLR* 32, Mar. 2002.

32. Stevens v. Contra Costa Reg'l Med. Ctr., Cal., settled before filing, Dec. 17, 2001. 17 *PNLR* 46, Apr. 2002.

33. Doe v. Roe, Md., confidential court, docket no., and date. 17 *PNLR* 48, Apr. 2002.

34. Solomon v. Desert Valley Hosp., Inc., Cal., San Bernardino County Super. Ct., No. VCV017352, Sept. 10, 2001. 17 *PNLR* 51, Apr. 2002.

35. Palmer v. South Ala. Nursing Homes, Inc., Ala., Mobile County Cir. Ct., No. CV002775, Dec. 14, 2001. 17 *PNLR* 52, Apr. 2002.

36. Johnson v. Weiss Mem'l Hosp., Ill., Cook County Cir. Ct., No. 01 L 6581, Mar. 13, 2002. 17 *PNLR* 66, May 2002.

37. Doe v. Roe, N.C., confidential court and docket no., Dec. 18, 2001. 17 *PNLR* 66, May 2002.

38. Huckaby v. Lake Pointe Partners, LTD., Tex., Rockwall County 382d Jud. Dist. Ct., No. 1-00-592, Dec. 14, 2001. 17 *PNLR* 67, May 2002.

39. Doe v. Roe, N.C., confidential court and docket no., Jan. 2002. 17 *PNLR* 68, May 2002.

40. Nunn v. Galen of Ky., Inc., Ky., Jefferson County Cir. Ct., No. 97-CI-05753, Oct. 1, 2001. 17 *PNLR* 69, May 2002.

41. Moore v. Allegheny Univ. Hosp.-City Ave., Pa., Phila. County C.C.P., No. 980602267, Jan. 14, 2002. 17 *PNLR* 70, May 2002.

42. Doe v. Roe, Md., Baltimore City Cir. Ct., confidential docket no., June 14, 2001. 17 *PNLR* 71, May 2002.

43. Doe v. Roe, Cal., Los Angeles County Super. Ct., confidential docket no., Dec. 2001. 17 *PNLR* 71, May 2002.

44. Boze v. Universal Nursing Servs. *Ltd.,* Fla., Hernando County Cir. Ct., No. H-27-CA-2001-1706, Mar. 21, 2002. 17 *PNLR* 104, July 2002.

45. M.N. v. Variety Children's Hosp., Fla., Dade County Cir. Ct., No. 98-16750 CA 06, Dec. 19, 2001. 17 *PNLR* 108, July 2002.

46. Washington v. Kings Daughters Hosp., Miss., Washington County Cir. Ct., No. C197-0130, Mar. 28, 2002. 17 *PNLR* 110, July 2002.

47. Mays v. Palestine Principal Healthcare L.P., Tex., Anderson County 349th Jud. Dist. Ct., No. 4744, Feb. 22, 2002. 17 *PNLR* 111, July 2002.

48. Jones v. Chicago HMO Ltd. Of Ill., 730 N.E.2d 1119 (2000).

49. Horizon/CMS Healthcare Corp. v. Auld, 34 S.W.3d 887 (2000).

50. Restatement (Second) of the Law of Agency §219 (1958).

51. In re Triss, 2002 WL 1271492 (La.App. 4 Cir., 2002).

52. Cavico, Frank J., and Cavico, Nancy M. (1995) The Nursing Profession in the 1990s: Negligence and Malpractice Liability. 43 Clev. St. L. Rev. 557.

53. Babcock, Linda, and Pogarsky, Greg. (1999) Damages Caps and Settlement: A Behavioral Approach. 28 Journal of Legal Studies 341.

54. Black's Law Dictionary 396 (8th ed. 2005).

CHAPTER 6
NCLEX-RN Preparation

Patricia Kelly, Maureen T. Marthaler

OBJECTIVES

Upon completion of this chapter, the reader should be able to:

1. Outline preparation for the National Council of State Boards of Nursing Licensure Examination for Registered Nurses (NCLEX-RN).

2. Relate factors associated with NCLEX-RN performance.

3. Outline components of organizing a review to prepare for NCLEX-RN.

Anwar will be graduating from his nursing education program in two months. He plans to focus his current efforts on preparing to take the NCLEX-RN Licensure Examination. He knows that three areas of examination preparation are possessing the knowledge, being adept at CAT testing, and controlling test anxiety.

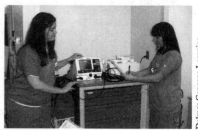

How should he prepare for the examination?

Where should he focus?

How can he decrease his test anxiety?

A new graduate from an educational program that prepares RNs will take the National Council of State Boards of Nursing Licensure Examination for Registered Nurses (NCLEX-RN). NCLEX-RN is taken after graduation and prior to practice as an RN. It is wise to schedule the exam date soon after graduation. The examination is given across the United States at professional testing centers. Graduates submit their credentials to the state board of nursing in the state in which licensure is desired. After the state board accepts the graduate's credentials, the graduate can schedule the examination. Successful completion of this examination ensures a basic level of safe nursing practice to the public. This is essential to working as a professional RN. The examination follows a test plan formulated on four categories of client needs that RNs commonly encounter. Integrated processes include the nursing process, caring, communication and documentation, and teaching/learning. These are integrated throughout the four major categories of client needs (NCSBN, 2010). See Table 6-1. This chapter discusses preparation for NCLEX-RN.

NCLEX-RN

All RN candidates must answer a minimum of 75 items on the NCLEX-RN examination. There is a maximum number of 265 items on the exam. Six hours are allocated to the student for the exam including instructions and all rest breaks. Computerized Adaptive Testing (CAT), which uses computer technology and measurement theory, is used for the exam. Test items go through an extensive review process before they can be used on the examination. In addition to multiple choice items, candidates may be administered items written in alternate formats,

TABLE 6-1
NCLEX-RN TEST PLAN

Client Needs Tested	Percent of Test Questions
Safe and effective care environment:	
Management of care	16–22%
Safety and infection control	8–14%
Health promotion and maintenance:	
Psychosocial integrity	6–12%
Physiological integrity	6–12%
Basic care and comfort	6–12%
Pharmacological and parenteral therapies	13–19%
Reduction of risk potential	10–16%
Physiological adaptation	11–17%

From *NCLEX-RN Test Plan, effective April 2010*. Retrieved March 1, 2010, from www .NCSBN.org

e.g., multiple response, fill-in-the-blank, drag and drop, or hot spots. All item types may include multimedia such as charts, tables, graphics, sound, and video. With CAT, each candidate's examination is unique because it is assembled interactively as the examination proceeds. Computer technology selects items to administer from a large item pool. After the candidate answers an item, the computer calculates the candidate's ability estimate based on all of the candidate's previous answers. The next item is then chosen that measures the candidate's ability most precisely in the appropriate test plan category. This process is repeated for each item creating an examination tailored to the candidate's knowledge and skills while fulfilling all NCLEX-RN Test Plan requirements. The examination continues with items selected and administered in this way until a pass or fail decision is made. More information about the NCLEX examination, including CAT methodology, items, the candidate bulletin and Web tutorials, is listed on the NCSBN Web site at www.ncsbn.org.

SAMPLE QUESTIONS

The various formats for test questions are illustrated here.

Test Question 1—Fill in the blank

A man underwent an exploratory laparoscopy yesterday. Calculate his intake and output for an eight-hour period.

Intake	**Output**
IV-0.9% NS at 125 mL/hr	Foley urine output 850 mL
PO-1 ounce ice chips	NG tube-200 mL
IVPB 30 mL Q8H mL	
Intake _____	Output _____

Test Answer 1

Intake = 1,060 mL; Output = 1,050 mL

125 mL/hr (125 mL × 8 hr) is 1,000 mL; 1 ounce of ice chips is 30 mL;

IVPB 30 mL Q8H (30 mL × 1) is 30 mL for a total of 1,060 mL.

Output is 850 mL urine and 200 mL of nasogastric drainage for a total of 1,050 mL.

Test Question 2—Multiple Response

A woman has been diagnosed with cervical cancer and will be undergoing internal radiation in addition to surgery. The nurse is planning her nursing care. Check all that are appropriate in maintaining a safe environment.

_____ Minimizing staff contact with the patient

_____ Utilizing required shielding

_____ Encouraging staff to stay at the foot of the bed or at the entrance to the room

_____ Wearing isolation gowns when entering the room (Stein, 2005)

Test Answer 2

"Minimizing staff contact with the patient" should be checked. Radiation is cumulative. Limiting the amount of time with the patient limits the nurse's exposure to radiation.
"Utilizing required shielding" should be checked. Shielding made of heavy metal decreases the amount of radiation exposure.

"Encouraging the staff to stay at the foot of the bed or at the entrance to the room" should be checked. Exposure decreases with greater distance from the radiation source.

"Wearing isolation gowns when entering the room" should not be checked. Isolation gowns offer no protection against radiation (Stein, 2005).

Test Question 3—Multiple-choice, single answer questions

The lab results of a 68-year-old male reveal an elevated titer of *Helicobacter pylori*. Which of the following statements, if made by the nurse, indicates an understanding of this data?

1. "Treatment will include antibiotics."
2. "No treatment is necessary at this time."
3. "This result indicates a gastric cancer caused by the organism."
4. "Surgical treatment is indicated."

Test Answer 3

1. *Helicobacter pylori* is the organism believed to cause most peptic ulcers. The organism has multiple flagella allowing it to move through the mucous layer of the stomach, thereby interfering with the local protection of the gastric mucosa against acid. Treatment with antibiotics and an acid-suppressing drug is indicated to prevent chronic atrophic gastritis (a predisposition to cancer).
2. Treatment with antibiotics and acid-suppressing drugs is indicated when the *H. pylori* titer is elevated.
3. An elevated *H. pylori* does not by itself indicate cancer. An untreated infection predisposes to cancer. Cancer is diagnosed with a biopsy. Most people with elevated *H. pylori* do not have gastric cancer.
4. Surgical treatment of an ulcer is indicated when medical approaches fail and the client has a bleeding ulcer (Stein, 2005).

Test Question 4—Fill in the blank

A medication is ordered to be given at 6 cc/hr. The solution is 20,000 mg/500 cc. How many mg per hour will that deliver to the patient?

Test Answer 4

$$\frac{20,000 \text{ mg}}{500 \text{ cc}} = \frac{40 \text{ mg}}{1 \text{ cc}}$$
$$= 40 \times 6$$
$$= 240 \text{ mg per hour}$$

Test Question 5—Use of Hot spot

Identify the height of the fundus at 22 weeks on this picture.

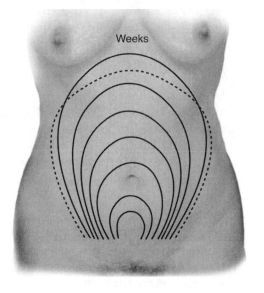

Test Answer 5

The fundus is located at this site at 22 weeks.

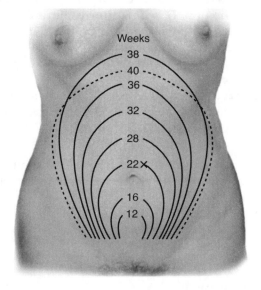

Test Question 6—Arrange responses in correct order (drag and drop)

Arrange these steps in the correct order to insert a Foley catheter.

1. Check integrity of Foley balloon.
2. Attach drainage bag to bed.
3. Cleanse meatus.
4. Spread the labia.
5. Insert the Foley.

Test Answer 6

1. **Check integrity of Foley balloon.**
4. **Spread the labia.**
3. **Cleanse meatus.**
5. **Insert the Foley.**
2. **Attach drainage bag to bed.**

EXIT EXAMINATIONS

Many nursing programs administer an examination to students at the completion of their nursing program. New graduates will want to review their performance on any of these exit exams because these results will help identify their weaknesses and focus their review sessions. Students who examine their feedback from an exit exam have important information that can help them focus their review for the NCLEX.

PREDICTORS OF NCLEX-RN SUCCESS

Several predictors have been identified in research studies as being associated with performance on the NCLEX examination. Some of these predictors are identified in Table 6-2. Students can work to strengthen any weaknesses in their predictors as they prepare for NCLEX-RN.

NCLEX-RN REVIEW BOOKS AND COURSES

In preparing to take the NCLEX, the new graduate may find it useful to focus preparation in three areas: NCLEX knowledge review, NCLEX test question practice, and test-anxiety control. Review books often include nursing content, sample test questions, or both. They frequently include computer software disks with test questions. The test questions may be arranged in the NCLEX book by clinical content area, or they can be presented in one or more comprehensive examinations covering all areas of the NCLEX. Listings of these review books are available at www.amazon.com. It is helpful to use several of these books and software

> **TABLE 6-2**
> *PREDICTORS OF NCLEX SUCCESS*
>
> - HESI Exit Exam
> - Verbal SAT score
> - ACT score
> - High-school rank and grade point average (GPA)
> - Undergraduate nursing program GPA
> - GPA in science and nursing theory courses
> - Competency in American English language
> - Reasonable family responsibilities or demands
> - Absence of emotional distress
> - Critical-thinking competency

programs when preparing for the NCLEX. Focus on NCLEX review sources developed in the past three years.

Some resources for reducing test anxiety include a Tame test anxiety CD-ROM by Richard Driscoll (2003) and two books: *Taking the anxiety out of taking tests* by Susan Johnson (2000) and *Test anxiety prevention* by Rosenthal and Rosenthal (2004).

NCLEX review courses are also available. Brochures advertising these programs are often sent to schools and are available in many sites nationwide. The quality of these programs can vary, and students may want to ask former nursing graduates and faculty for recommendations. An NCSBN-sponsored review course and a test question of the week are available at www.learningext.com.

KEEP YOUR PATIENTS SAFE 6-1

You are responsible for being the nurse you want to be. To do this, set your goals and monitor and evaluate them regularly. Gather data on the following indicators of being a professional nurse and add to the list, as appropriate. What other goals have you added?
- Develop skills and education specific to the unit I am working on.
- Pass the NCLEX-RN exam.
- Monitor data so that I am up to date on evidence-based care for my patients.
- Monitor data that my patients are satisfied, pain-free, and feel cared about.

(continues)

Keep Your Patients Safe 6-1 *(continued)*

- Monitor data that my patients are complication-free and have no nurse-sensitive outcomes.
- Offer professional nursing service to my patients and my community.
- Give and receive professional respect to and from health care team.
- Speak up about the important role that nurses play in preventing patient complications.
- Network with other professionals.
- Participate on professional committees at work.
- Communicate assertively with the health care team.
- Receive professional salary and benefits.
- Take good care of myself and work for professional and personal balance.
- Continue my education, for example, certification, formal education, continuing education, and so on.
- Join my professional organization.
- Dress like a professional.
- Communicate pride in being a nurse.

REAL WORLD INTERVIEW

My best advice to anyone preparing for the NCLEX is to take lots of practice tests. I answered close to 1,500 questions in preparation, and I feel it did me a world of good. I kept my nursing textbooks handy, and when I ran into something I didn't know, I looked it up.

Amanda Meadows, RN, BSN
Chicago, Illinois

KNOWLEDGE, ANXIETY MANAGEMENT, AND TEST-TAKING SKILL

Successful test performance requires nursing knowledge, anxiety management, and test-taking skill. Knowledge of the test content is the first critical element. Students gain knowledge of nursing as the result of a course of nursing study. Nursing students attend either a two-year associate degree nursing program, a three-year diploma nursing program, or a four-year baccalaureate nursing program to gain the knowledge needed to satisfactorily complete the NCLEX-RN.

Anxiety management such as visualization and relaxation techniques before and during the test is the second element of successful test performance. Plan to use any or all of the following to control your anxiety level:
- Positive thinking
- Guided imagery, which requires using your imagination to create a relaxing sensory scene on which to concentrate
- Breathing exercises
- Relaxation exercises
- Relaxation audio tapes (Stein, 2005)
- Enjoying hard peppermint candy

Test-taking skills are the final critical element needed for successful test completion. Strategies to improve test-taking skills include practicing 60 test questions daily from different NCLEX-RN review books, CDs, and online NCLEX review sites such as www.delmarlearning.com, until performance is satisfactory on all areas of the NCLEX exam. Note that successful students often practice 60 questions daily in their knowledge weakness areas until their performance improves. Practicing 60 questions daily for 30 days exposes students to 1,800 questions ($60 \times 30 = 1,800$). Use the results of an exit exam or comprehensive exam to guide you in your selection of test questions. Practice using the ARKO (Action, Reword, Key, Options) and ABC-Safe methods discussed later in this chapter as you review the test questions.

ORGANIZING YOUR REVIEW

In preparing for NCLEX, identify your strengths and weaknesses. If you have taken an exit exam, note any content strength and weakness areas in your exam results. Look carefully at the elements of the NCLEX-RN test plan (refer to Table 6-1). Complete a self-analysis of NCLEX-RN preparation needs (Table 6-3), and establish a schedule that permits you to cover completely all the material to be learned. Note any nursing program course or clinical content areas in which you scored below a grade of B. Purchase one or more of the NCLEX review books. It is useful to review questions developed by different authors. Review content in the review books in any of your weak content areas. Take a comprehensive exam in the review book or on the computer software disk and analyze your performance. Try to answer as many questions correctly as you can. As you study, be sure to actually practice taking the examinations. Do not just jump ahead to the answer section until you have completed the examination. Completing the examination in this way may improve your examination performance.

Next, after you have completed the comprehensive examination, review the answers and rationales for any weak content areas and take

TABLE 6-3
SELF-ANALYSIS OF NCLEX-RN PREPARATION NEEDS

Anxiety level (circle) 1 2 3 4 5 6 7 8 9 10
Weak content areas identified on NCLEX Test Plan in Table 6-1, exit exam, or comprehensive exam, etc.

_____

_____

_____

Nursing courses below grade of B: _____
Predictors from Table 6-2 _____

_____

Weak content areas identified in leading causes of death in the United States:
- Mental health, for example, schizophrenia, bipolar disorders, anxiety, personality disorders, suicide, eating disorders, abuse, and so on _____

_____

- Women's health, for example, antepartum care, intrapartum care, postpartum care, newborn care, and so on _____

_____

- Adult health, for example, cancer, myocardial infarction, diabetes, pneumonia, HIV, hepatitis, cholecystectomy, CVA, nephrectomy, renal failure, thyroidectomy, shock, appendectomy, and so on

_____

- Children's health, for example, leukemia, cardiovascular surgery, fractures, cancer, diabetes, asthma, Wilm's tumor, cleft palate, and so on

_____

Weak content areas identified in any of the following areas:
- Therapeutic communication
- Growth and development (developmental milestones and toys)
- Management, delegation, referrals, and priority setting
- Medications
- Defense mechanisms
- Immunizations
- Diagnostic tests and laboratory values

Organize Your Review

Your study schedule could look like the following, depending on the feedback from your self-analysis:
Day 1: Practice 60 adult health test questions. Score the test, analyze your performance, and review test question rationales and content weaknesses. Practice deep breathing, relaxation exercises, and positive thinking, as needed.

(continues)

Table 6-3 *(continued)*

Day 2: Practice 60 women's health test questions. Repeat above process.
Day 3: Practice 60 children's health test questions. Repeat above process.
Day 4: Practice 60 mental health test questions. Repeat above process.
Day 5: Continue with knowledge review and test question practice in all weak knowledge areas. Practice deep breathing, relaxation exercises, and positive thinking. Continue this process until you are doing well in all areas.
Study when you are most alert!

another comprehensive exam. Repeat this process until you are doing well in all clinical content areas and in all areas of the NCLEX examination plan. Use methods of memory improvement that will work for you. Mnemonic devices, where a letter represents the first letter of each item in a sequence, are an effective means of recalling information as you study. For instance, one mnemonic device is "it is OK to have your blood tested while on anticoagulants." This is a memory device to assist you in remembering the antidote for Coumadin overdose—that is, the antidote for Oral Coumadin is Vitamin K (OK). Remembering this can help you eliminate the antidote for the other anticoagulant, Intravenous Heparin. Heparin's antidote is Protamine Sulfate.

Mental imagery is the technique of forming pictures in your mind to help you remember details of the sequence of events, such as the administration of an injection. Another technique is practicing self-recitation to improve your study habits. Reciting to yourself the material being learned will promote retention of the information being studied. Focus on the information you identified in your self-analysis of your NCLEX-RN preparation needs.

Do a general review of the common patient diseases, medications, diagnostic tests, and nursing procedures in each major nursing content area, as well as defense mechanisms, communication tips, and growth and development. These strategies will assist you in conquering the three areas necessary for successful test-taking—anxiety management, knowledge, and test-taking skills.

Organize the material so that you will be able to review all the need-to-know information within the allotted study time period. Your schedule should have allowed you to complete your review so you can close your books and do something relaxing on the night before the examination.

Nutrition, Sleep, and Wardrobe.   You will function best if you are well nourished. Plan to eat three well-balanced meals a day for at least three days prior to the examination. Be careful when choosing the food you consume within 24 hours of the examination. Avoid foods that will make you thirsty or cause intestinal distress. Minimize the potential of a full bladder midway through the examination by limiting the amount of fluids you drink and by allowing sufficient time at the test site to use the bathroom before entering the room.

Plan to allow sufficient time in your schedule the week before the examination to provide yourself with the minimum sleep you need to function effectively for at least three days prior to the examination. Plan your wardrobe ahead of time. Shoes and clothes that fit you comfortably and suit the temperature will not distract your thought processes during the examination. Your clothes for the test day should be ready to wear by the night before the examination. If you wear glasses or contact lenses, take along an extra pair of glasses. If you are taking medications on a regular basis, continue to do so during this period of time. Introduction of new medications should be avoided until after completion of the examination (Stein, 2005).

CASE STUDY 6-1

Analyze your learning needs based on Table 6-3. Use Table 6-4 to identify your best time to practice NCLEX questions and review content. Complete the schedule for the next week. When is your best time to study? Is it morning or evening? Review the question of the week each Monday and note the NCLEX review course at the NCSBN site, www.learningext.com.

NCLEX AND MEDICATION GUIDES

Table 6-5 has some more tips on reviewing for NCLEX. Table 6-6 is a Medication Study Excerpt to aid you in your NCLEX preparation. Use these tools as a starting point in your review for NCLEX.

ARKO STRATEGIES AND ABC-SAFE-COMFORT TIPS

When you are presented with a difficult test question, use these ARKO test-taking strategies and ABC-Safe-Comfort tips to improve your test performance. Use ARKO strategies as follows:

- **A**: Is the question stem asking you to take **A**ction or take no **A**ction?
- **R**: **R**eword the question.

	M	T	W	R	F	S	S
TABLE 6-4 ***ORGANIZING YOUR PLANS FOR NCLEX STUDY***							
8–9							
9–10							
10–11							
11–12							
12–1							
1–2							
2–3							
3–4							
4–5							
5–6							
6–7							
7–8							
8–9							
9–10							

- **K**: Identify any **K**ey words in the question stem.
- **O**: Eliminate incorrect answer **O**ptions.

Apply this ARKO strategy to the following test question:

What should the nurse do first for a patient with a spinal cord injury who complains of a headache?
   A. Empty the patient's bladder.
   B. Assess the patient's pupils.
   C. Take the patient's blood pressure.
   D. Administer a beta-adrenergic blocker.

Apply the ARKO strategy to the previous question.
   A: Stem asks for nurse to take **A**ction, i.e., insert a Foley catheter.
   R: **R**eword the question, as follows: What is a priority nursing action for a patient with a spinal cord injury who has a headache?
   K: **K**ey words are "first," "spinal cord injury," and "headache."
   O: Note the following as you eliminate incorrect options:
      Option A may be useful if the blood pressure is elevated, as a full bladder can trigger autonomic dysreflexia.

TABLE 6-5
SELECTED NCLEX TIPS

- Remember Maslow's Hierarchy of Needs. Physical needs are met first, for example, airway, breathing, circulation (ABCs) threats
  - Airway
    - Altered level of consciousness (LOC)
    - Unconscious
    - Foreign object in airway
  - Breathing
    - Asthma
  - Circulation
    - Cardiac arrest
    - Shock
- Safety needs are met second, for example, safety and infection control threats
  - Confusion
  - Tuberculosis
  - Isolate noninfectious patients from infectious patients
- Comfort and healing needs and teaching needs are met after physical ABC and safety needs are met. Don't choose a test question answer that gives the patient comfort or healing or meets teaching needs before the patient's physical ABC and safety needs have been met.
- Remember the nursing process—Assess your patient first; then plan, implement, and evaluate.
- Keep all your patients safe: for example, airway open; siderails up; IV access line in place on unstable patient; monitor vital signs, pulse oximeter, cardiac rhythm, and urine output, as needed.
- Know delegation guidelines for RNs, LPN/LVNs, and NAP. Observe the Five Rights of Delegation—that is, the right task, the right circumstance, the right person, the right direction/communication, and the right supervision. See Chapter 2.
  - The RN assures quality care of all patients, especially patients with complex needs. RNs delegate care of stable patients with predictable outcomes.
  - The RN uses patient care data such as vital signs, collected either by the nurse or others, to make clinical judgments. The RN continuously monitors and evaluates patient care and delegates care involving standard, unchanging procedures to LPN/LVNs and NAP.
  - The RN makes appropriate referrals to community resources.
  - The RN never delegates patient Assessment, Teaching, Evaluation (ATE), or judgment.
  - LPN/LVNs can perform medication administration, sterile dressings, Foley insertions, and so on.

(continues)

Table 6-5 (continued)

- In some states, LPN/LVNs can insert IVs, pass nasogastric tubes, and so on, with documented competency.
- NAP can perform basic care, for example, vital sign measurement, bathing, transferring, ambulating, communicating with patients, and stocking supplies.
- In some states, NAP can perform venipuncture, do blood glucose tests, insert Foley catheters, and so on, with documented competency.
- Avoid mixing patients with an infection, for example, bacterial sepsis, with patients who have decreased immunity, for example, a patient with AIDS, diabetes, on steroids, the very young, the very old, and so on.
- In answering test questions, do the following:
  - When choosing priorities, choose the first answer reflecting what you would do if you were alone and could only do one thing at a time. Don't think that one RN will do one thing, and another RN will do another thing.
  - Assume you have the health care provider's order for any possible choices. NCLEX is usually looking for the correct nursing action, not the medical action.
  - Assume you have perfect staffing, plenty of time, and all the necessary equipment for any possible test question choices. Choose the answer that indicates the best nursing care possible.
  - Assume you are able to give perfect care "by the book." Don't let your personal clinical experience direct you to choose a test answer that is less than high-quality care.
  - Remember to care for the patient first and then check the equipment.
- Know the most common adult, maternal-child, and psychological health care disorders. For each disorder, know the medications, laboratory and diagnostic tests, procedures, and treatments commonly used.
- Know common medications (see Table 6-6).
- Know common laboratory norms, for example, sodium, potassium, blood sugar, complete blood count, white cell count, hemoglobin, hematocrit, prothrombin time, partial thromboplastin time, international normalized ratio (INR), arterial blood gas (ABG), cardiac enzymes, digoxin level, dilantin level, lithium level, blood urea nitrogen (BUN), creatinine, uric acid, and specific gravity of urine.
- Know communication techniques—look for answers that give patients support and allow them to keep talking and verbalize their concerns and problems. Be their comforting nurse, not their therapist. Avoid advice.
- Know common food choices included in special diets, for example, low sodium diet, diabetic diet, and so on.

(continues)

Table 6-5 *(continued)*

- Know common food choices for potassium, protein, sodium, vitamin K, calcium, etc.
- Know the defense mechanisms.
- Know growth and development, such as the developmental tasks for each childhood stage, toys for each childhood stage, and so on.
- Know immunization schedules.
- Prepare with the following:
  - ○ Anxiety control and relaxation techniques
  - ○ Regular exercise
  - ○ Positive thinking and avoidance of negative people
  - ○ Avoidance of thought distortions (see Chapter 3)
  - ○ Visualize your name with "RN" next to it on your name tag
- Remember—you graduated from an accredited nursing program. You can do it!

TABLE 6-6
MEDICATION STUDY EXCERPT

Complete/add to this as you study for NCLEX-RN
General Tips
1. Drowsiness Guidelines: If drowsiness is listed in the following chart, consider the need to monitor airway, level of consciousness (LOC), blood pressure (BP), pulse (P), respirations (R), pulse oximetry, and cardiac rhythm. May need to have an IV line in place to assure emergency medication access and safeguard patient. Use siderails/fall precautions as needed. Patient may need to avoid driving and alcohol.
2. Drowsiness and changes in vital signs (VS) are a side effect of many medications given for their analgesic, antiemetic, antiseizure, tranquilizer, sedative/hypnotic, antihistamine, or antianxiety effects.
3. Blood Pressure (BP) Medication (Med) Guidelines: Note that if the drug is a cardiac or BP drug, use BP Med Guidelines, i.e., consider the need to monitor LOC, cardiac rhythm, BP, P, R, and pulse oximetry. May need to take note of postural hypotension and maintain fall precautions.
4. Many medications cause renal, liver, heart, brain, and/or bone marrow side effects. Monitor labs that reflect the functions of these organs. Check allergies.
5. Haldol, Ativan, and Cogentin mixture is often used PRN for restraints—try nonrestrictive approaches first.

(continues)

Table 6-6 *(continued)*

Category	Prefix or Suffix	Examples	Patient Implications
Phenothiazine	zine	Promethazine (Phenergan)	Drowsiness Guidelines
Antiemetic Antipsychotic Antianxiety		Fluphenazine (Prolixin)-IM	Extrapyramidal (EPS) symptoms, Parkinsonism, akathisia (restless), dystonia (jerky movement, spasms, check airway), tardive dyskinesia (involuntary movements)
			Teach patient to report irreversible early EPS symptoms
Benzodiazepines	Azepam	Diazepam (Valium);	Drowsiness Guidelines
Tranquilizer Hypnotic Antianxiety Antiseizures Anesthetic	Aze	Lorazepam (Ativan); Clonazepam (Klonopin); Alprazolam (Xanax); Midazolam (Versed)	Check for habituation; taper dose when discontinued
			Monitor bone marrow, liver, and kidney laboratory tests
			Versed used for short-term sedation—monitor closely
			Romazicon (Flumazenil) reverses sedative effect of benzodiazepines
Anticoagulant	Parin	Heparin (Antidote is Protamine Sulfate)	Monitor bleeding, e.g., stool, gums, urine, bruising
			For Heparin, check PTT. Give Heparin IV to get PTT to 1.5–2 times the control time.
Anticoagulant		Coumadin (Warfarin) (Antidote is Vitamin K)	Monitor bleeding, e.g., stool, gums, urine, bruising
			Check PT/INR (desirable INR range is 2.0–3.0 for patients on coumadin)
Angiotensin Converting Enzyme (ACE inhibitor) Antihypertensive	Pril	Lisinopril (Zestril) Enalapril (Vasotec) Ramipril (Altace)	BP Med Guidelines

(continues)

Table 6-6 *(continued)*

Category	Prefix or Suffix	Examples	Patient Implications
Angiotensin Receptor Blocking Agents Antihypertensive	Sartan	Telmisartan (Micardis) Irbesartan (Avapro) Losartan (Cozaar)	BP Med Guidelines
Beta-adrenergic Blockers Antihypertensive Antianginal	Olol	Metaprolol (Lopressor) Propanolol (Inderal)	BP Med Guidelines Monitor for bronchospasm, bradycardia
Antihypertensive	Pres	Clonidine (Catapres) Hydralazine (Apresoline)	BP Med Guidelines
Calcium Channel Blockers Antihypertensive	Pine	Nifedipine (Procardia) Amlodipine (Norvasc)	BP Med Guidelines
Antihyperlipidemic	Vastatin	Lovastatin (Mevacor) Atorvastatin (Lipitor)	Check renal, liver, and cholesterol labwork Muscle cramping is side effect
Diuretic	Ide	Lasix (Furosemide)	Monitor intake and output Check potassium level
Potassium		Potassium electrolyte	Give IVPB slowly—use IV pump for infusions Potassium can kill if given quickly Be sure patient has adequate urine output and normal creatinine level before giving

(continues)

Table 6-6 *(continued)*

Category	Prefix or Suffix	Examples	Patient Implications
Anti-infectives	Mycin Cin	Gentamycin (Garamycin) Vancocin (Vancomycin)	Check allergy, monitor for ototoxicity, seizures, blood dyscrasias, nephrotoxicity, rash
			Monitor peak and trough, BUN, and creatinine
Anti-infectives	Ceph Cef	Cephalexin (Keflex) Ceftriaxone (Rocephin)	Check allergy, monitor liver and renal lab tests
Antiviral	Vir	Zidovudine (Retrovir) Acyclovir (Zovirax)	Monitor for nausea and vomiting, tremors, confusion
			Check liver and renal lab tests
Non Steroidal Anti-inflammatory Drug (NSAID)	Cox	Celecoxib (Celebrex)	Tinnitus/GI bleed
			Monitor platelets, renal function, BUN, and creatinine
Steroids Anti-inflammatory Many anti-inflammatory uses for conditions such as CVA, asthma, arthritis, etc.	One	Decadron (Dexamethasone) Prednisone (Deltasone) Methylprednisolone (Solu-Cortef, Depo-Medrol)	Monitor seven "Ss": sex, sadness, stress, sight, susceptibility, sugar, sodium
			Decreases sex (hormones), stress (inflammatory response), sight (cataracts), and potassium
			Increases sadness (mood), susceptibility (infection, ulcers), sugar (hyperglycemia), sodium (edema), and osteoporosis
			Wean off steroids to avoid adrenal crisis and shock

(continues)

Table 6-6 *(continued)*

Category	Prefix or Suffix	Examples	Patient Implications
Histamine (H2) Receptor Antagonists	Tidine	Ranitidine (Zantac)	
Inhibits gastric acid secretion		Famotidine (Pepcid)	
Proton Pump Inhibitors	Prazole	Esomeprazole(Nexium)	
Used for erosive gastro-esophageal reflux disease (GERD)		Pantoprazole (Protonix)	
		Rabeprazole (Aciphex)	
		Lansoprazole (Prevacid)	
Miotic Eye Drops		Pilocarpine	Constricts the pupil and reduces intraocular pressure
Mydriatic Eye Drops		Atropine	Dilates the pupil

OTHER MEDICATIONS			
Antipsychotic	Antiarrhythmic	Antidepressant	Mood Stabilizer
Zyprexa Seroquel Haldol Prolixin Abilify Risperdal (Risperdal M melts in the mouth for patients who are med avoiders)	Amiodarone (Cordarone); Norpace (Disopyramide); Rythmol (Propafenone); Tambocor (Flecainide); Betapace (Sotalol) Monitor BP, P, electrolytes, especially K and Mg—Monitor Heparin and cardiac rhythm	Celexa Cymbalta Lexapro Zoloft Paxil Prozac Remeron (older patient) Drowsiness guidelines	Lithium (know levels) , BP guidelines Depakote (hair loss) Tegretol

(continues)

Table 6-6 *(continued)*

OTHER IMPORTANT MEDICATIONS
Atropine, Benadryl, Cogentin, Digoxin, Epinephrine, Insulin, Lasix, Lactulose, Magnesium Sulfate, Morphine, Neurontin, Pitocin, Synthyroid, Isoniazid, Rifampin, Ethambutol, Pyrazinamide, Rhogam, Zyloprim, etc.
From Kelly, P., & Hernandez, G. Unpublished manuscript.

Option B does not give us useful information about this patient.

Option C is useful to assess blood pressure for autonomic dysreflexia.

Option D will reduce blood pressure, but stem does not say blood pressure is elevated.

The correct answer is C.

ABC-Safe-Comfort Tips.   As you review a test question, it is helpful to review Maslow's Hierarchy of Needs and use the ABC-Safe-Comfort tips. Assess your patient's ABCs, then assess his or her Safety, and, finally, after these are assured, assess your patient's Comfort and Healing needs and then consider any Teaching needs. Remember this order when prioritizing your nursing actions:

A – Airway

B – Breathing

C – Circulation

Safety

Comfort and Healing

Teaching

Apply these tips to this test question:

The nurse is unable to obtain a pedal pulse on Doppler examination of the cold painful leg of a patient who has just been admitted with a fractured femur. What is the priority intervention for this patient?

A. Give Morphine, as ordered.

B. Teach the patient cast care.

C. Notify the health care provider.

D. Comfort the patient and keep the leg elevated.

Apply ABC-Safe-Comfort tips to the question's options.

A. Comfort can be given with the pain medication, but this is an emergency. Call the health care provider. Comfort care is done after ABC and Safety are assured.

B. Teaching is done after ABC-Safe-Comfort is assured.

C. Patient has an absent pulse on Doppler and a cold, painful leg—this is an emergency! Patient's arterial circulation cannot be occluded long before there is permanent damage to tissues.

D. Patient is not safe or comforted if there is no arterial circulation to leg. Comfort care is done after ABC and Safety are assured.

Answer is C.

Recall that NCLEX often wants you to take all nursing actions before calling the health care provider. In an emergency, however, do not hesitate to call the health care provider. Always recall that Maslow's Hierarchy of Needs directs us to monitor our patient's ABCs and then keep them Safe. After this is done, we can offer Comfort and Healing and Teach our patients.

REAL WORLD INTERVIEW

A dean that I know talks about the fact that she failed what was called in those days "the boards." She tells her students that it was the most traumatic event of her life (or at least one of the most traumatic events). When you have given it "your all" to complete a nursing curriculum, you want to be a successful NCLEX candidate. The HESI Exit Exam can help you achieve that goal. Look at your score printout and review any subject area that has a HESI score of less than 850. Remember, HESI scores are NOT percentage scores, but research data indicate that those who have HESI scores of 850 or above have a 94% probability of passing the NCLEX-RN.

Susan Morrison, PhD, RN
Former President, Health Education Systems, Inc. (HESI)
Houston, Texas

EVIDENCE FROM THE LITERATURE

Citation: Gordon, S., & Nelson, S. (2006). *Moving beyond the virtue script in nursing in the complexities of care.* Ithaca, NY: ILR Press.

Discussion: Author discusses the concept that images of hearts and angels and the emphasis on caring and health in nursing trivialize what is in fact highly skilled knowledge work that addresses the important role of nurses in care of the sick. The author states that hospital administrators, politicians, and the public won't expand the effort to decode nursing. Nurses must articulate a vivid picture of how nurses as a profession protect their patients. Nursing is facing a crisis because potential recruits

(continues)

Evidence from the Literature *(continues)*

don't understand that nurses prevent fatal complications and assess and monitor their patients using knowledge-based scientific care. An emphasis on caring devalues the nursing role, attracting the wrong recruits and driving practitioners from the role. Many nurses are tough-minded professionals who value their technical and practical expertise. They are often dismissed as uncaring. The author asks, isn't using technology and knowledge to prevent complications an act of caring?

Implications for Practice: Nurses must monitor nursing-sensitive indicators and demonstrate the lifesaving role nurses play with their patients using knowledge-based scientific practice. This process begins with passing the NCLEX.

CASE STUDY 6-2

Nirmala is a Nursing Assistive Personnel (NAP) who has just completed her nursing education program. She is caring for Patty Homan in Room 2506 and Bobbie Anderson in Room 2512 today. As she finishes the shift, Nirmala says to the RN she is working with, "I am so afraid that I will not pass NCLEX. Do you have any suggestions for me?" What three areas of test preparation should the RN mention in her answer?

 # REVIEW QUESTIONS

1. The nurse is planning care for a three-month-old infant immediately postoperative following placement of a ventriculoperitoneal shunt for hydrocephalus. The nurse needs to do which of the following?
   A. Monitor neurological status and infection.
   B. Maintain infant in an upright position.
   C. Begin formula feedings when infant is alert.
   D. Pump the shunt to assess for proper function.

2. A 16-year-old presents to the emergency department. The triage nurse finds that this teenager is legally married and signed the consent for treatment form. What would be the appropriate INITIAL action by the nurse?
   A. Refuse to see the patient until a parent or legal guardian can be contacted.
   B. Withhold treatment until telephone consent can be obtained from the spouse.

    C. Refer the patient to a community pediatric hospital emergency room.

    D. Assess and treat in the same manner as any adult patient.

3. A patient with a pulmonary embolism has the following arterial blood gases: PaO_2 – 60 mm Hg, PCO_2 – 32 mm Hg, pH – 7.45, HCO_3 – 22. Based on this data, what should be the FIRST nursing action?

    A. Review other lab data

    B. Notify the physician

    C. Administer oxygen

    D. Calm the patient

4. As the nurse interviews the parents of a child with asthma, it is a PRIORITY to ask about which of the following?

    A. Household pets

    B. New furniture

    C. Lead-based paint

    D. Plants such as cactus

5. When the nurse becomes aware of feeling reluctant to interact with a manipulative patient, the BEST action by the nurse is to do which of the following?

    A. Discuss the feeling of reluctance with an objective peer or supervisor.

    B. Limit contacts with the patient to avoid reinforcing the manipulative behavior.

    C. Confront the patient regarding the negative effects of his or her behavior on others.

    D. Develop a behavior modification plan that will promote more functional behavior.

6. While obtaining the history of a two-week-old infant during the well-baby exam, the nurse finds that the neonatal screening for phenylketonuria (PKU) was done when the infant was less than 24 hours old. It is a PRIORITY for the nurse to do which of the following?

    A. Schedule the infant for a repeat test in two weeks.

    B. Obtain a repeat blood test at this point.

    C. Contact the hospital of birth for the results.

    D. Document that the test results are pending.

7. The patient was given 20 mg of Lasix (furosemide) PO at 10 a.m. What information would be essential for the nurse to include at the change of shift report?

    A. The patient lost two pounds.

    B. The patient's potassium level is 4 mEq/dl.

    C. The patient's urine output was 1,500 cc in five hours.

    D. The patient is to receive another dose of Lasix at 10 p.m.

8. Which of the following instructions would be most appropriate as the nurse provides discharge teaching to the parents of a 15-month-old child with Kawasaki Disease who has received immunoglobulin therapy?
   A. High doses of aspirin should be continued for some time.
   B. Complete recovery is expected within several days.
   C. Active range of motion exercises should be done frequently.
   D. The measles, mumps, and rubella vaccine should be delayed.

9. Lactulose (Chronulac) has been prescribed for a patient with advanced liver disease. Which of the following assessments would the nurse use to evaluate the effectiveness of this treatment?
   A. An increase in appetite
   B. A decrease in fluid retention
   C. A reduced ammonia level
   D. A reduction in jaundice

10. The nurse is reinforcing teaching to a 24-year-old woman receiving acyclovir (Zovirax) for a Herpes Simplex Virus Type 2 infection. The nurse should instruct the patient to do which of the following?
    A. Complete the entire course of the medication for an effective cure.
    B. Begin treatment with acyclovir at the onset of symptoms of recurrence.
    C. Stop treatment if she thinks she may be pregnant to prevent birth defects.
    D. Continue to take prophylactic doses for at least five years after the diagnosis.

11. The nurse is teaching a patient with non–insulin-dependent diabetes mellitus about the prescribed diet. The nurse should teach the patient to do which of the following?
    A. Maintain previous calorie intake.
    B. Keep a candy bar available at all times.
    C. Reduce carbohydrate intake to 25% of total calories.
    D. Keep a regular schedule of meals and snacks.

12. Two hours after the normal spontaneous vaginal delivery of a woman who is gravida 4 para 4, the nurse notes that the fundus is boggy and displaced slightly above and to the left of the umbilicus. The appropriate initial nursing action is to do which of the following?
    A. Assess lochia for color and amount.
    B. Monitor pulse and blood pressure.
    C. Call the physician immediately.
    D. Ask the woman to empty her bladder.

13. Which nursing intervention will be MOST effective in helping a withdrawn patient to develop relationship skills?
    A. Offer the patient frequent opportunities to interact with you.
    B. Remind the patient frequently to interact with other patients.
    C. Assist the patient to analyze the meaning of her behavior.
    D. Identify other patients for her who have similar problems.

14. As the nurse takes a history of a three-year-old with neuroblastoma, what comments by the parents require follow-up and are consistent with the diagnosis?
    A. "The child has been listless and has lost weight."
    B. "She only passes small amounts of dark yellow urine."
    C. "Clothes are becoming tighter across her abdomen."
    D. "We notice muscle weakness and some unsteadiness."

 APPLY YOUR SKILLS

1. Set up a group to study for NCLEX with several of your friends. Arrange to meet to discuss how your NCLEX review is going. Have each member of the group buy an NCLEX review book from a different publisher. Practice answering questions for one to two hours daily. Don't mark your answers in your review book. Share your review books with each other to increase your exposure to various authors' test questions.

2. Go to www.ncsbn.org. Review the detailed test plan for students there. Do you see any content areas that you should review more carefully?

3. Practice test-taking using all of the test question formats identified in this chapter. Use different NCLEX review books. Do you find any of the formats more difficult than others?

4. Review your test scores from either an exit exam or a comprehensive exam from an NCLEX review book. Do you identify any areas for further review?

5. Review the Medication Study Excerpt in Table 6-6. Become comfortable with the prefix/suffix for different categories to increase your ability to recognize medications. Review all the medications in the medication study excerpt as you prepare for NCLEX-RN. Pay particular attention to the actions, side effects, and nursing implications as you review and add them to the excerpt.

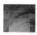

EXPLORING THE WEB

1. Review NCLEX review books at www.amazon.com. How many different books published in the past three years did you see on the topic of NCLEX review?

2. Go to www.ncsbn.org. Bookmark it and note what you see there. Explore the site.

3. Go to www.learningext.com. NCSBN's review for the NCLEX is offered through this NCSBN learning extension. This self-paced, online review features NCLEX-style questions, interactive exercises, topic-specific course exams, and a diagnostic pretest that can help you develop a personal study plan. Visit this Web site every Monday to see its new NCLEX-RN test question samples.

REFERENCES

Driscoll, R. (2003). *Tame test anxiety: Powerful stress reduction means more gain with less pain.* Lodi, NJ: Westside Publishing.

Gordon, S., & Nelson, S. (2006). *Moving beyond the virtue script in nursing in the complexities of care.* Ithaca, NY: ILR Press.

Johnson, S. (2000). *Taking the anxiety out of taking tests.* New York, NY: Barnes & Noble books.

Kelly, P., & Hernandez, G. Unpublished manuscript.

NCLEX-RN Examination. Test plan for the National Council Licensure Examination for Registered Nurses. (2010). Chicago, IL: National Council of State Boards of Nursing. Retrieved March 1, 2010, from www.ncsbn .org/1287.htm

Nightingale, F. (1872). *Florence Nightingale to her nurses: A selection from Miss Nightingale's addresses to probationers and nurses of the Nightingale Scholl at St. Thomas's Hospital* [p. 1; Address in May 1872]. London: Macmillan.

Rosenthal, H. G., & Rosenthal, R. G. (2004). *Test anxiety prevention.* London, UK: Routledge Pub.

Stein, A. M. (2005). *NCLEX-RN review* (5th ed.). Clifton Park, NY: Delmar Cengage Learning.

SUGGESTED READINGS

Aucoin, J. W., & Treas, L. (2005). Assumptions and realities of the NCLEX-RN. *Nursing Education Perspective, 26*(5), 268–271.

Bondmass, M. D., Moonie, S., & Kowalski, S. (2008). Comparing NET and ERI standardized exam scores between baccalaureate graduates who pass or fail the NCLEX-RN. *International Journal of Nursing Education Scholarship, 5*(1), 16.

Bonis, S., Taft, L., & Wendler, M. C. (2007). Strategies to promote success on the NCLEX-RN: An evidence-based approach using the ACE Star Model of Knowledge Transformation. *NLN Nursing Education Perspectives, 28*(2), 82–87.

Crow, C. S., Handley, M., Morrison, R. S., & Shelton, M. M. (2004). Requirements and interventions used by BSN programs to promote and predict NCLEX-RN success: A national study. *Journal of Professional Nursing, 20*(3), 174–186.

Cunningham, H., Stacciarini, J. M., & Towle, S. (2004). Strategies to promote success on the NCLEX-RN for students with English as a second language. *Nurse Educator, 29*(1), 15–19.

Davenport, N. C. (2007). A comprehensive approach to NCLEX-RN success. *NLN Nursing Education Perspectives, 28*(1), 30–33.

DiBartolo, M. C., & Seldomridge, L. A. (2005). A review of intervention studies to promote NCLEX-RN success of baccalaureate students. *Nurse Educator, 30*(4), 166–171.

DiBartolo, M. C., & Seldomridge, L. A. (2008). A review of intervention studies to promote NCLEX-RN success of baccalaureate students. *Computers Informatics Nursing, 26*(5 Suppl), 78–83S.

Downey, T. A. (2008). Predictive NCLEX success with the HESI Exit Examination: Fourth annual validity study. *Computers Informatics Nursing, 26*(Suppl. 5), 35S–36S, author reply 36S–38S.

English, J. B., & Gordon, D. K. (2004). Successful student remediation following repeated failures on the HESI exam. *Nurse Educator, 29*(6), 266–268.

Frith, K. H., Sewell, J. P., & Clark, D. J. (2005). Best practices in NCLEX-RN readiness preparation for baccalaureate student success. *Computers Informatics Nursing, 23*(6), 322–329.

Frith, K. H., Sewell, J. P., & Clark, D. J. (2008). Best practices in NCLEX-RN readiness preparation for baccalaureate student success. *Computers Informatics Nursing, 26*(Suppl. 5), 46S–53S.

Giddens, J., & Gloeckner, G. W. (2005). The relationship of critical thinking to performance on the NCLEX-RN. *Journal of Nursing Education, 44*(2), 85–90.

Griffiths, M. J., Papastrat, K., Czekanski, K., & Hagan, K. (2004). The lived experience of NCLEX failure. *Journal of Nursing Education, 43*(7), 322–325.

Lyons, E. M. (2008). Examining the effects of problem-based learning and NCLEX-RN scores on the critical-thinking skills of associate degree nursing students in a Southeastern Community College. *International Journal of Nursing Education Scholarship, 5*(1), 21.

McDowell, B. M. (2008). KATTS: A framework for maximizing NCLEX-RN performance. *Journal of Nursing Education, 47*(4), 183–186.

Morrison, S., Free, K. W., & Newman, M. (2008). Do progression and remediation policies improve NCLEX-RN pass rates? *Computers Informatics Nursing, 26*(Suppl. 5), 67S–69S.

Morton, A. M. (2008). Improving NCLEX scores with structured learning assistance. *Computers Informatics Nursing, 26*(Suppl. 5), 89S–91S.

Nibert, A. T., & Young, A. (2008). A third study on predicting NCLEX success with the HESI exit exam. *Computers Informatics Nursing, 26*(Suppl. 5), 21S–27S.

Nibert, A. T., Young, A., & Adamson, C. (2008). Predicting NCLEX success with the HESI Exit Exam: Fourth annual validity study. *Computers Informatics Nursing, 26*(Suppl. 5), 28S–34S.

Sifford, S., & McDaniel, D. M. (2007). Results of a remediation program for students at risk for failure of the NCLEX exam. *NLN Nursing Education Perspectives, 28*(1), 34–36.

Sitzman, K. L. (2007). Diversity and the NCLEX-RN: A double-loop approach. *Journal of Transculture Nursing, 18*(3), 271–276. Review.

Spurlock, D. R., Jr., & Hunt, L. A. (2008). A study of the usefulness of the HESI Exit Exam in predicting NCLEX-RN failure. *Journal of Nursing Education, 47*(4), 157–166.

Sutherland, J. A., Hamilton, M. J., & Goodman, N. (2007). Affirming At-Risk Minorities for Success (ARMS): Retention, graduation, and success on the NCLEX-RN. *Journal of Nursing Education, 46*(8), 347–353.

Uyehara, J., Magnussen, L., Itano, J., & Zhang, S. (2007). Facilitating program and NCLEX-RN success in a generic BSN program. *Nursing Forum, 42*(1), 31–38.

GLOSSARY

Accountability   Being responsible and answerable for actions or inactions of self or others in the context of delegation.

Activity log   Time management tool that can assist the nurse in determining how both personal and professional time is used.

Administrative law   Laws that deal with protection of the rights of citizens.

Anger   A universal, strong feeling of displeasure that is often precipitated by a situation that frustrates or prevents a person from attaining a goal.

Assignment   The downward or lateral transfer of both the responsibility and accountability of an activity from one individual to another.

Attending   Activity involving active listening.

Authority   The right to act or to command the action of others.

Blaming   Finding fault or error; this occurs when a response lacks respect for others' feelings.

Civil law   Law that governs the relationship between individuals.

Clarifying   Communication that becomes clear through the use of such techniques as restating and questioning.

Communication   An interactive process that occurs when a person (the sender) sends a verbal or nonverbal message to another person (the receiver) and receives feedback.

Competence   The ability of the nurse to act with and integrate the knowledge, skills, values, attitudes, abilities, and professional judgment that underpin effective and quality nursing and are required to practice safely and ethically in a designated role and setting.

Confronting   To work jointly with others to resolve a problem or conflict.

Constitution   A set of basic laws that specifies the powers of the various segments of the government and how these segments relate to each other.

Critical thinking   Indicates "thinking about your thinking while you're thinking in order to make your thinking better."

Delegation   The transfer of responsibility for the performance of an activity from one individual to another while retaining accountability for the outcome.

False imprisonment   Occurs when individuals are incorrectly led to believe they cannot leave a place.

Good samaritan laws   Laws that have been enacted to protect the health care professional from legal liability for actions rendered in an emergency when the professional is giving service without pay.

Indirect patient care   Activities often necessary to support the patient and his or her environment, and which only incidentally involve direct patient contact.

Malpractice   A nurse's wrongful conduct in discharge of his or her professional duties or failure to meet standards of care for the profession, which results in harm to another individual entrusted to the nurse's care.

Negligence   The failure to provide the care a reasonable person would ordinarily provide in a similar situation.

Nursing judgment   The process by which nurses come to understand the problems, issues, or concerns of clients; to attend to salient information; and to respond to client problems in concerned and involved ways.

Pareto principle   Principle stating that 20% of focused effort results in 80% of desired outcomes or results, or conversely that 80% of unfocused effort results in 20% of desired outcomes results.

Public law   Consists of constitutional law, criminal law, and administrative law and defines a citizen's relationship with government.

Responding   Verbal and nonverbal acknowledgment of the sender's message.

Responsibility   Obligations involved when one accepts an assignment.

Supervision   Providing of guidance or direction oversight, evaluation, and followup by the licensed nurse for the accomplishment of a nursing task delegated to assistive personnel.

Time management   A set of related common-sense skills that helps nurses use their time in the most effective and productive way possible.

INDEX

Note: Page numbers followed with t refer to Tables

239